Avascular Necrosis of the Carpal Bones: Etiologies and Treatments

Editors

CHARLES A. DALY
MITCHELL A. PET

HAND CLINICS

www.hand.theclinics.com

Consulting Editor
KEVIN C. CHUNG

November 2022 • Volume 38 • Number 4

ELSEVIER

1600 John F. Kennedy Boulevard ● Suite 1800 ● Philadelphia, Pennsylvania, 19103-2899

http://www.theclinics.com

HAND CLINICS Volume 38, Number 4
November 2022 ISSN 0749-0712, ISBN-13: 978-0-323-98751-6

Editor: Megan Ashdown
Developmental Editor: Hannah Almira Lopez

Hand Clinics (ISSN 0749-0712) is published quarterly by Elsevier Inc., 360 Park Avenue South, New York, NY 10010-1710. Months of publication are February, May, August, and November. Business and Editorial Offices: 1600 John F. Kennedy Blvd., Ste. 1800, Philadelphia, PA 19103-2899. Customer Service Office: 3251 Riverport Lane, Maryland Heights, MO 63043. Periodicals postage paid at New York, NY and at additional mailing offices. Subscription price is $444.00 per year (domestic individuals), $1060.00 per year (domestic institutions), $100.00 per year (domestic students/residents), $506.00 per year (Canadian individuals), $1081.00 per year (Canadian institutions), $568.00 per year (international individuals), $1081.00 per year (international institutions), $256.00 (international students/residents), and $100.00 (Canadian students/residents). Foreign air speed delivery is included in all *Clinics* subscription prices. All prices are subject to change without notice. **POSTMASTER:** Send address changes to *Hand Clinics*, Elsevier Health Sciences Division, Subscription Customer Service, 3251 Riverport Lane, Maryland Heights, MO 63043. Customer Service (orders, claims, online, change of address): Elsevier Health Sciences Division, Subscription **Customer Service, 3251 Riverport Lane, Maryland Heights, MO 63043. Tel: 1-800-654-2452 (U.S. and Canada); 314-447-8871 (outside U.S. and Canada). Fax: 314-447-8029. E-mail: journalscustomerservice-usa@elsevier.com (for print support); journalsonlinesupport-usa@elsevier.com (for online support).**

Reprints. For copies of 100 or more of articles in this publication, please contact the Commercial Reprints Department, Elsevier Inc., 360 Park Avenue South, New York, New York 10010-1710. Tel.: 212-633-3874; Fax: 212-633-3820; E-mail: reprints@elsevier.com.

Hand Clinics is covered in *MEDLINE/PubMed (Index Medicus), Current Contents/Clinical Medicine, EMBASE/Excerpta Medica,* and *ISI/BIOMED.*

Contributors

CONSULTING EDITOR

KEVIN C. CHUNG, MD, MS
Charles B.G. de Nancrede Professor of
Surgery, Professor of Plastic Surgery and
Orthopaedic Surgery, Chief of Hand Surgery,
Department of Surgery, Section of Plastic
Surgery, Michigan Medicine, Assistant Dean
for Faculty Affairs, Associate Director of Global
REACH, University of Michigan Medical
School, Comprehensive Hand Center,
University of Michigan, The University of
Michigan Health System, Ann Arbor, Michigan,
USA

EDITORS

CHARLES A. DALY, MD
Assistant Professor, Director of
Musculoskeletal Quality, Department of
Orthopaedic Surgery, Division of Upper
Extremity Surgery, Medical University of South
Carolina, Charleston, South Carolina, USA

MITCHELL A. PET, MD
Assistant Professor, Department of Plastic and
Reconstructive Surgery, Washington
University in St. Louis, St Louis, Missouri, USA

AUTHORS

JEREMY A. ADLER, MD
Orthopaedic Surgery Resident, UChicago
Medicine and Biological Sciences, Chicago,
Illinois, USA

**GREGORY I. BAIN, PhD, MBBS, FRACS,
FA(ORTHO)A**
Professor, Department of Orthopaedic Surgery
and Trauma, Flinders Medical Centre, Flinders
University, Bedford Park, South Australia,
Australia; Professor, Hand and Upper Limb
Surgery, Flinders University, Adelaide, South
Australia, Australia

**SIMON F. BELLRINGER, MBBS, BSc, FRCS
(Tr&Orth)**
Department of Orthopaedic Surgery and
Trauma, Flinders Medical Centre, Bedford
Park, South Australia, Australia

CATHLEEN CAHILL, MD
Orthopaedic Surgery Resident, UChicago
Medicine and Biological Sciences, Chicago,
Illinois, USA

COURTNEY CARLSON STROTHER, MD
Resident, Department of Orthopaedic Surgery,
Mayo Clinic, Rochester, Minnesota, USA

JOSEPH CATAPANO, MD, PhD
Division of Plastic and Reconstructive Surgery,
St. Michael's Hospital, University of Toronto,
Toronto, Ontario, Canada

KEVIN C. CHUNG, MD, MS
Charles B.G. de Nancrede Professor of
Surgery, Professor of Plastic Surgery and
Orthopaedic Surgery, Chief of Hand Surgery,
Department of Surgery, Section of Plastic
Surgery, Michigan Medicine, Assistant Dean
for Faculty Affairs, Associate Director of Global
REACH, University of Michigan Medical
School, Comprehensive Hand Center,
University of Michigan, The University of
Michigan Health System, Ann Arbor, Michigan,
USA

MEGAN CONTI MICA, MD
Associate Professor of Orthopaedic Surgery
and Rehabilitation Medicine, UChicago

Medicine and Biological Sciences, Chicago, Illinois, USA

CHARLES A. DALY, MD
Assistant Professor, Director of Musculoskeletal Quality, Department of Orthopaedic Surgery, Division of Upper Extremity Surgery, Medical University of South Carolina, Charleston, South Carolina, USA

JOHN C. DUNN, MD
William Beaumont Army Medical Center, Texas Tech University Health Sciences Center El Paso, El Paso, Texas, USA; Uniformed Services University of the Health Sciences, Bethesda, Maryland, USA

MATTHEW M. FLORCZYNSKI, FRCSC, MD, MS
Hand Surgery Fellow, Section of Plastic Surgery, Department of Surgery, University of Michigan Medical School, Ann Arbor, Michigan, USA

ALEXANDER REED GRAF, MD
Department of Orthopedic Surgery, Division of Upper Extremity Surgery, Emory University, Emory Orthopaedics & Spine Center, Atlanta, Georgia, USA

CARL M. HARPER, MD
Department of Orthopaedic Surgery, Boston, Massachusetts, USA

JAMES P. HIGGINS, MD
The Curtis National Hand Center, MedStar Union Memorial Hospital, Baltimore, Maryland, USA

MINHAO HU, BClinSc, MD, MSurg
Department of Plastic and Reconstructive Surgery, Flinders Medical Centre, Adelaide, South Australia, Australia

ALEXANDER LAUDER, MD
Department of Orthopedics, University of Colorado School of Medicine, Aurora, Colorado, USA; Department of Orthopedic

Surgery, Denver Health Medical Center, Denver, Colorado, USA

W. CHARLES LOCKWOOD, MD
Department of Orthopedics, University of Colorado School of Medicine, Aurora, Colorado, USA; Department of Orthopedic Surgery, Denver Health Medical Center, Denver, Colorado, USA

SIMON B.M. MACLEAN, MBChB, FRCS(Tr&Orth), PGDipCE
Consultant Orthopaedic and Upper Limb Surgeon, Department of Orthopaedic Surgery, Tauranga Hospital, Tauranga, North Island, New Zealand; Department of Orthopaedic Surgery, Tauranga Hospital, Bay of Plenty, New Zealand

MITCHELL A. PET, MD
Assistant Professor, Department of Plastic and Reconstructive Surgery, Washington University in St. Louis, St Louis, Missouri, USA

BRENT B. PICKRELL, MD
Department of Orthopedic Surgery, Massachusetts, USA

NICHOLAS PULOS, MD
Assistant Professor, Department of Orthopaedic Surgery, Mayo Clinic, Rochester, Minnesota, USA

KASHYAP K. TADISINA, MD
Department of Plastic and Reconstructive Surgery, Washington University in St. Louis, St Louis, Missouri, USA

ERIC R. WAGNER, MD
Emory University, Department of Orthopedic Surgery, Division of Upper Extremity Surgery, Emory Orthopaedics & Spine Center, Atlanta, Georgia, USA

MATTHEW E. WELLS, DO
William Beaumont Army Medical Center, Texas Tech University Health Sciences Center El Paso, El Paso, Texas, USA

CONTENTS

Avascular necrosis is a complicated, multifactorial disease with potentially devastating consequences. Although the underlying root cause is a lack of appropriate vascular perfusion to affected bone, there are often varying patient-specific, anatomic-specific, and injury-specific predispositions. These factors generally fall into 3 categories: direct vascular disruption, intravascular obliteration, or extravascular compression. The initial stages of disease can be insidiously symptomatic because edematous bone marrow progresses to subchondral collapse and subsequent degenerative arthritis. Although much of the current literature focuses on the femoral head, other common areas of occurrence include the proximal humerus, knee, and the carpus. The low-incidence rate of carpal avascular necrosis poses a challenge in establishing adequately powered, control-based validated treatment options, and therefore, optimal surgical management remains a continued debate among hand surgeons. Appreciation for expectant fracture healing physiology may help guide future investigation into carpal-specific causes of avascular necrosis.

The vascular anatomy of the wrist is vital in the development of multiple disorders at the carpus. Understanding this vascular network may prevent iatrogenic injury to the blood supply and can be used by surgeons through vascularized bone grafts. Multiple surgical techniques take advantage of the vascular network. This article reviews the blood supply of the distal radius, ulna, and carpal bones and its clinical implications.

In the now 110 years that have passed since Kienböck first published his seminal description of lunate osteonecrosis, improvements in imaging technology and surgical technique have provided a better understanding of Kienböck disease pathogenesis and treatment. However, the precise etiology, natural history, and optimal treatment remain controversial. Future studies examining the genetics behind the disease and large-scale prospective studies comparing treatment options represent the next step in improving our understanding of this rare and complex phenomenon.

Kienböck disease (KD) involves osseous, vascular, and chondral aspects of the lunate and wrist. We present our theories on the etiology and pathogenesis of the condition based on basic science models, seminal literature, personal case experience, and kinematic observations of the Kienböck wrist. Three phenotypes of Kienböck disease occur, and each tends to have different morphology, rates of progression, and disease pattern. The lunate fracture in KD is well-recognized but different fracture types can occur. Dynamic assessment of the Kienböck wrist allows assessment of the complex kinematics of KD. Disease onset and progression require a "perfect storm" of risk factors.

Robert Kienböck described radiographic changes associated with idiopathic lunate osteonecrosis in 1910. The radiographic progression of this eponymous condition has been well-described to progress from normal radiographs, to lunate sclerosis, lunate collapse, proximal capitate migration, scaphoid flexion, and pancarpal arthritis. Diagnosing early stages of the disease without radiographic changes presented a challenge. As imaging modalities have evolved, diagnosis has become possible with MRI. Although numerous classification systems exist, the Lichtman classification and the Bain arthroscopic grading system have become widely used. This article outlines the available classification systems and aims to highlight when each may be useful in patient management.

The algorithm and rationale described is a reflection of our own surgical experience for this challenging disorder and can be compared with other publications. Our algorithm has evolved from treatment of a large volume of patients with Kienböck disease in a referral practice. However, it is limited to the management that we have found logical, effective, and within our scope of experience. The treatment guidelines for our specialty as a whole will evolve as our understanding of the etiology and our ability to quantify efficacy improves.

Various osteotomies, core decompression, and denervation all have demonstrated favorable outcomes in treatment of Kienböck disease. Given the rarity of this disease, there is a dearth of high-level comparative studies to direct treatment. In this article, the authors review the current literature surrounding these techniques, and provide summary recommendations for the procedure choice.

Of the many treatments for Kienböck disease, only lunate revascularization procedures provide a direct mechanism for reversing the process of osteonecrosis. Owing to the redundant blood supply of the distal radius and carpus, pedicled flaps are versatile solutions for patients with bone loss but intact cartilage. With the advent of free vascularized flaps, the indications for lunate revascularization procedures are expanding. These flaps can be used when the articular cartilage has been compromised and are suitable options to restore native anatomy in patients previously thought to have unreconstructible disease.

Jeremy A. Adler, Megan Conti Mica, and Cathleen Cahill

Kienbock's disease is a progressive condition characterized by lunate collapse, carpal instability, and eventually perilunate arthritis. Etiology is likely multifactorial, including vascular and anatomic or osseus causes. In cases of advanced disease, disabling pain, limited motion, and decreased grip strength may be present. The preferred treatment options for the nonreconstructable wrist are proximal row carpectomy (PRC), total wrist arthrodesis, and total wrist arthroplasty (TWA). In the following chapter, we will discuss various surgical options for patients with advanced Kienbock's disease.

Eric R. Wagner and Alexander R. Graf

Wrist arthroscopy represents the most recent development in the diagnosis and treatment of Kienböck disease. Through direct visualization of lunate and adjacent carpal articulations, a more accurate diagnosis can be obtained and, ultimately, a more precise treatment decision. Treatments that are based on bypassing, fusing, or excising "nonfunctional" articulations can be done with less morbidity than traditional open techniques by using arthroscopy. Given the minimal capsular and soft tissue scarring, this potentially improves early pain and functional recovery. Although technically demanding, long-term outcomes studies have shown that the benefits of an arthroscopic approach may be worth the learning curve.

Simon F. Bellringer, Simon B.M. MacLean, and Gregory I. Bain

Video content accompanies this article at http://www.hand.theclinics.com.

The term Preiser's disease typically is used to describe idiopathic avascular necrosis of the scaphoid, but there have been a number of putative etiologies considered. It is rare and the natural history is not fully understood. Management of the condition should be based on patient factors as well as the stage of disease with regard to the scaphoid and the surrounding wrist. This chapter appraises the available evidence and aims to provide the reader with a framework to manage this rare condition.

Brent B. Pickrell and Carl M. Harper

Outside of Preiser and Kienbock disease, avascular necrosis (AVN) of the remaining carpal bones is a rare cause of wrist pain and disability with a natural history that is incompletely understood. At present, much of the available clinical information exists in the form of isolated case reports or small case series. Although reported surgical treatment options are numerous, there is a dearth of comparative studies and long-term outcomes data with which to guide management.

HAND CLINICS

Preface

Avascular Necrosis of the Carpal Bones: Etiologies and Treatments

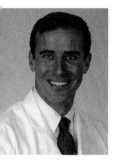 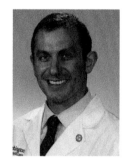

Charles A. Daly, MD   Mitchell A. Pet, MD
Editors

Part of the richness of hand surgery is its inclusion of many rare and puzzling pathologic conditions that occasionally test the surgeon's diagnostic skills, cognitive flexibility, and technical facility. This adds to both the allure and the challenge of our great field. Avascular processes of the carpus perfectly epitomize this truth. In our opinion, this is an exciting field wherein gaps in our understanding of the pathophysiology and natural history of this disease constellation has fostered immense surgical creativity and iterative innovation.

In some ways, the uncertainty surrounding Kienbock and Preiser disease (and their even rarer counterparts affecting the remaining carpus) makes these clinical challenges enjoyable to treat and inspiring to research. However, especially in the era of algorithms and evidence-based medicine, the absence of a single underlying logic that underpins current clinical practice can leave both patients and clinicians feeling adrift. Different pathomechanical and physiologic suppositions spawn treatment that may seem to be entirely unrelated to each other and a body of clinical evidence that can be impossible to reconcile. It is our recognition of this issue that prompted us to choose this topic as the focus of this *Hand Clinics* issue.

Herein, we aim to summarize the best available evidence supporting our understanding of avascular processes of the carpus. Recognizing that the evidence is insufficient to completely guide clinical practice, this issue also necessarily includes experience and theory-based practice recommendations from thought-leaders in the field. While it is our hope that this issue will serve as a useful guide to management, our enthusiasm is tempered by the understanding that the current corpus of information summarized herein is still incomplete, though developing and evolving rapidly. We fully expect, and are excited to be a part of, the evolution of our understanding of this disease process over the years and decades to come.

Charles A. Daly, MD
Department of Orthopaedics and Physical Medicine, Medical University of South Carolina, Clinical Sciences Building, CSB, 96 Jonathan Lucas Street, MSC Code: 708, Charleston, SC 29425, USA

Mitchell A. Pet, MD
Department of Plastic and Reconstructive Surgery, Washington University in St. Louis, Center for Advanced Medicine, Plastic and Reconstructive Surgery Center, 4921 Parkview Place, Floor: 6, Suite: G, St. Louis, MO 63110, USA

E-mail addresses:
dalyc@musc.edu (C.A. Daly)
mpet@wustl.edu (M.A. Pet)

Hand Clin 38 (2022) ix
https://doi.org/10.1016/j.hcl.2022.03.010
0749-0712/22/© 2022 Published by Elsevier Inc.

hand.theclinics.com

Pathophysiology of Avascular Necrosis

Matthew E. Wells, DO[a,b,*], John C. Dunn, MD[a,b,c]

KEYWORDS

- Pathophysiology • Avascular necrosis • AVN • Carpal bones • Osteochondritis dissecans
- Osteonecrosis • Preiser • Kienbock

KEY POINTS

- Avascular necrosis is a complicated, multifactorial disease with a predisposition for certain osseous areas throughout the skeletal system, including the carpal bones.
- Although primarily seen in the lunate (Kienböck disease) and scaphoid (Preiser disease), avascular necrosis has now been described in all carpal bones.
- There are many proposed causes of avascular necrosis; however, each cause generally falls into one of the 3 categories: (1) direct vascular disruption, (2) intravascular obliteration, or (3) extravascular compression.
- There is a paucity of literature investigating the pathophysiology of carpal-specific avascular necrosis; however, many prior investigations can be used for extrapolation purposes. The most compelling carpal-specific investigations have focused on vascular anatomy.
- Further mechanistic investigation involving thrombosis formation and fracture healing physiology may help guide future investigation into carpal-specific causes of avascular necrosis.

INTRODUCTION

Avascular necrosis (AVN) is defined by the loss of appropriate vascular perfusion resulting in necrosis of osteocytes and bone marrow. AVN may occur throughout the body, but presents most commonly in anatomic locations such as the hip, jaw, and carpus. There are variety of identified factors that may predispose to AVN, although the reasons for occurrence of AVN remain incompletely understood. These include, but are not limited to trauma, repetitive forceful sport activities, corticosteroid use, gout, alcohol consumption, scleroderma, systemic lupus erythematosus, chemotherapy, mucopolysaccharidosis, and other genetic causes.[1–21]

Although there are many different potential causes, the final mechanism is always critical ischemia. The initial edematous bone marrow can be insidiously symptomatic and is a primary cause for early pain in AVN.[22] Later stages of AVN involve subchondral collapse and degenerative arthritis with subsequent chronic, debilitating pain. The goals of treatment are to improve pain, reduce the risk of progressive degenerative disease, and maximize functional outcomes.[23]

There has been considerable investigation into the causality, pathoanatomic changes, and treatment modalities in AVN of larger joints such as the femoral head, proximal humerus, or knee.[24–27] However, there is a paucity of research into AVN specific to the carpal bones likely due to the overall lower incidence as compared with aforementioned anatomic regions. Although we believe that many of the concepts established in the hip literature are translatable to the carpus, it should not be assumed that everything found to be true in the hip is necessarily applicable to in the carpus. This review outlines the relevant studies regarding the pathophysiology of AVN and provides an overview of clinical relevance to the hand surgeon.

[a] William Beaumont Army Medical Center, El Paso, TX, USA; [b] Texas Tech University Health Sciences Center El Paso, El Paso, TX, USA; [c] Uniformed Services University of the Health Sciences, Bethesda, MD, USA
* Corresponding author. Department of Orthopaedic Surgery, William Beaumont Army Medical Center, 18511 Highlander Medics Street, Fort Bliss, TX 79918.
E-mail address: Matthew.Eric.Wells@gmail.com

Hand Clin 38 (2022) 367–376
https://doi.org/10.1016/j.hcl.2022.03.011
0749-0712/22/Published by Elsevier Inc.

Three Proposed Mechanisms of Avascular Necrosis

Although it is a given that osteocyte and marrow necrosis occurs as a consequence of impaired circulation, the pathogenic factors leading to this state of malperfusion are not obvious. Three major mechanisms of AVN have been proposed and are discussed throughout the literature. These are vascular disruption, intravascular obliteration, and interosseous extravascular compression[28] (**Fig. 1**). Although categorization of these causes is helpful for descriptive purposes, the reality is each case of AVN is likely multifactorial.

Vascular disruption

Vascular disruption entails direct interruption of the critical vascular structures supplying the carpal bones. This occurs most often as a result of direct trauma or repetitive microtrauma. Examples of this direct and singular traumatic vascular insult include devascularization of the proximal pole of the scaphoid after fracture or devascularization of the lunate after perilunate dislocation.[29] Chronic microtraumatic vascular insult is perhaps harder to conceptualize. Although this process cannot be directly observed, the epidemiology of Kienböck disease, which occurs predominantly in active manual laborers,[30,31] supports this idea of chronic microtraumatic AVN. Furthermore, the preponderance of specific anatomic patterns of the lunate and carpal articulations at large in the Kienböck population suggests this is well. Ulnar negative variance, relative lunate uncovering, and Viegas type 1[32] lunate morphology all may contribute to excessive and potentially microtraumatic loading across a relatively small proximal lunate articulation, and have been observed to maintain association with Kienböck disease.[33,34] Although this is infrequently discussed, this idea of microtraumatic insult as a cause of carpal AVN has been discussed by different groups with varying emphasis on vascular[35] or bony microtrauma.[34] In the authors' opinion, these are likely overlapping processes, especially given that bony microvascular and structural elements are so closely linked from an anatomic perspective.

Intravascular obliteration

As opposed to the action of external force on the carpal microvasculature, intravascular causes entail the occlusion of intact vascular channels. Occlusion may result from fat embolism, thrombosis, or thromboembolism. Fat emboli have been implicated in critical ischemia either through direct means or by triggering intravascular coagulation.[36] Glucocorticoids and dyslipidemia may promote fat embolus formation; however, overall fat embolism in the setting of carpal AVN is not well established. Thrombosis or thromboembolus as a cause for intraluminal vascular obliteration, and resultant AVN is most commonly encountered in patients with hematologic disorders such as sickle cell disease but can also be related to hereditary[37] or acquired[38,39] hypercoagulable states.

Interestingly, associations between AVN and abnormalities of the coagulation cascade have been observed apart from clinical thrombophilia. Jones and colleagues[40] observed that 37 of 45 (82%) patient with large joint osteonecrosis were found to have at least one laboratory marker of hypercoagulability compared with 30% of controls. This finding was supported in a similar study by Zalavras and colleagues[41] wherein 68 patients with AVN of the hip were found to have a substantial excess of coagulation abnormalities compared with control subjects.

Newer insights have looked into specific regulators of the coagulation cascade and their individual roles in the development of AVN, particularly alpha-2-macroglobulin (A2M). This plasma protein was originally identified on the luminal surfaces of endothelial cells of human arteries.[42] A2M serves many roles, one of which being enhancement of hemostasis through upregulation of the coagulation cascade.[43] A recent study investigated the histologic changes of AVN in corticosteroid-treated rats versus an age-matched control group.[44] Interestingly, the study found that glucocorticoid-exposed rats had a significant upregulation of A2M gene expression in comparison to the control group, which may serve as one (among others discussed below) explanation for the increased risk for AVN in patients who receive chronic corticosteroid treatments. A2M has also be implicated in cartilage degeneration[45] through binding and inactivation of osteoprotegrin[46] and may also inhibit the function of bone morphogenic protein (BMP)-1.[47]

Although these case-control and laboratory studies offer a considerable support to the supposition that abnormalities of intravascular coagulation contribute to the pathophysiology of AVN, it should be again pointed out that these studies included only patients with large joint AVN. The pertinence of intravascular obliteration to carpal AVN remains an area of promising investigation, however, cannot be viewed as a conclusively settled issue.

Intraosseous extravascular compression

Arlet and colleagues were the first to propose this intraosseous hypertension hypothesis based on their report of elevated bone marrow pressures in patients with femoral head AVN.[48] Subsequent

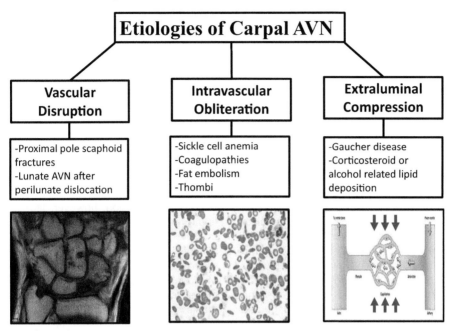

Fig. 1. Causes of carpal AVN.

confirmatory studies have displayed elevation in marrow pressures even before osteonecrosis was detectable.[49,50]

Intraosseous extraluminal compression has been thoughtfully and usefully conceptualized by Shah and colleagues using the model of a Starling resistor.[35] This resistor is described as compressible tubes (blood vessels) passing through a rigid-walled chamber (bone). The flow through these tubes (perfusion) is impacted by the extraluminal (intraosseous) pressure exerted upon their walls, and this pressure is in turn related to the volume of extraluminal material within this fixed space (**Fig. 2**). Therefore, in this model as additional tissue occupies the extraluminal space within a bone, the intraosseous pressure becomes elevated, and thereby decreases flow within the vascular channels traversing the bone. This conceptual model has been supported by Aaron and colleagues using contrast-enhanced magnetic imaging with gadolinium diethylene triamine pentaacetic acid to describe abnormalities in perfusion in subchondral bone in both animal and human models.[22] They found that venous outflow obstruction and blood flow stasis resulted intraosseous hypertension and subsequent physiologically relevant reductions in perfusion and PO_2.

Although the reasons for this observed hypertension are not completely understood, intraosseous lipid deposition and adipocyte hypertrophy have been observed. These mechanisms not only fit with the Starling resistor model outlined above[35] but also correlate with some of the empiric associations that have been observed to predispose to AVN. Both steroid and alcohol

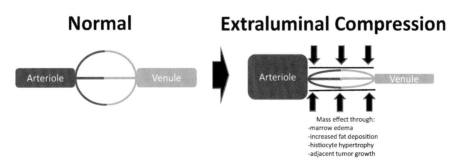

Fig. 2. The physiologic effect of extraluminal compression on intravascular pressures and subsequent perfusion.

exposure have been shown to cause increased affect lipid metabolism and adipocyte size.

With regard to corticosteroids, Wang and colleagues used animal models to show glucocorticoid administration leads to increased adipocyte size with a proportional decrease in intraosseous blood flow, which can be corrected by core decompression or statin therapy.[51–53] This finding not only supports the theory of extravascular compression but substantiates the rationale for core decompression of the lunate bone in cases of Kienböck disease.[54]

With regards to alcohol abuse, Matsuo and colleagues found that regular alcohol is associated with an increased risk of AVN, and that a clear dose–response relationship was evident.[55] Interestingly, in the same study, obesity was found to have no association with AVN, which underscores that generalized adiposity is not a marker for the excessive intraosseous lipid deposition and abnormal lipid metabolism, which are suspected to play a role in causing AVN by contributing to elevated intraosseous pressure. Aside from alcohol and corticosteroid exposure, other potential causes for critical marrow pressure elevation include, dyslipidemia, nitrogen bubbles, proliferation of histocytes in Gaucher disease, or bleeding from trauma.[23,28]

Vascular Anatomy as a Predisposing Factor for Carpal Avascular Necrosis

Insults to carpal bone perfusion occur in the context of normal or variant carpal vascular anatomy, which influences the likelihood that a given deficit will lead to necrosis. Osseous regions with tenuous blood supply have been established in multiple anatomic locations with subsequent similar risks for posttraumatic AVN.[56] Panagis

and colleagues were the first to categorize the carpal bones into different subgroups based on their overall vascular supply (**Table 1**).[57] The investigators used 25 cadaveric specimens to characterize the different intraosseous vascular anatomy within each carpal bone. This led to the classification of 3 groups that were at a descending risk for avascular necrosis (**Fig. 3**). The first group suffers from the greatest risk for AVN as they had vessels entering only one surface of the bone or the bone contained substantial areas dependent on a sole artery. The second group possesses an overall intermediate risk of AVN as they received multiple vessels for perfusion, however, lacked intraosseous anastomosis in a significant number of cadaveric models. The third group had the lowest risk of AVN as all models displayed 2 surfaces receiving blood supply, did not contain large areas of bone dependent on a single vessel, and all models displayed consistent intraosseous anastomosis patterns.

These vascular patterns help provide some insight into the overall incidence rates of AVN within the carpal bones. Lunate and scaphoid osteonecrosis, Kienböck disease and Preiser disease, respectively, are the 2 most commonly reported cases of avascular necrosis within the carpal bones. However, there have been case of avascular necrosis reported among all carpal bones.[1–20] The overall prevalence of these cases has been described in the following descending order: capitate, hamate, trapezium, trapezoid, triquetrum, and pisiform.[23]

Pathophysiology of Avascular Necrosis

AVN is often summarized as a failure of perfusion with resultant cell death. Although this is not necessarily incorrect, this simple explanation

Table 1
The classification of carpal bone vascularity as depicted by Panagis and colleagues

Classification of Intraosseous Vascularity of Carpal Bones	Group 1	Group 2	Group 3
Carpal Bones	Scaphoid, Capitate, Lunate (20%)	Trapezoid, Hamate	Trapezium, Triquetrum, Pisiform, Lunate (80%)
Definition	• Only 1 surface of bone with vascular penetration • Large intraosseous areas dependent on a sole artery	• 2 surface areas of bone with vascular penetration • Lacking intraosseous anastomosis	• 2 surface areas of bone with vascular penetration • Consistent intraosseous anastomosis
Risk of Avascular Necrosis	High	Intermediate	Low

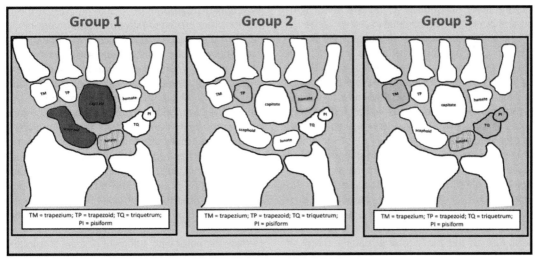

Fig. 3. The midline carpal bones are at increased risk for avascular necrosis compared with more peripheral carpal bones in accordance to the classification of carpal bone vascularity as depicted by Panagis and colleagues. TM, trapezium; TP, trapeziod; TQ, triquetrum; PI, pisiform.

omits some subtlety that is inherent to the process. Indeed, AVN does commence with a failure of perfusion, ostensibly related to one or more of the mechanisms cited above (**Table 2**). This results in early necrosis of hematopoietic cells and adipocytes, followed shortly thereafter by osteocyte necrosis.[35] This process is associated with marrow edema, which is often the earliest objective sign detectable in the clinical environment. This edema causes increased intraosseous pressure and worsens the situation of malperfusion and ischemic injury. As with any bodily injury, this cellular death event is met with a natural reparative process aimed to remove cellular debris and revascularize and rebuild what has been lost. New bone is laminated onto dead trabeculae, with partial resorption of the dead bone. In the subchondral region, the bone resorption inherent to this process exceeds new bone formation, resulting in a net loss of bone.[35] As such, the structural integrity of the subchondral trabeculae has compromised integrity and fails to adequately support the subchondral plate. This eventually results in subchondral fracture, collapse, and ultimately fragmentation. Altogether, it seems that vascular injury may lead to the early changes and initial step resulting in avascular necrosis. However, it is the bone remodeling that results in irreparable point of no return and eventual degenerative changes.[58–60]

In a 2016 publication, Drs Bain, Lichtman and colleagues expanded on this mechanism of trabecular failure (which again, has its origins in the hip literature) to explain specifically how it applied to Kienböck disease.[34] In their model, they propose repetitive and excessive loading of the lunate, which is often exacerbated by bony anatomic variants that increase load transmission across an "at risk" lunate. This results in edema of the adipocytes of the bone marrow, thereby causing increased intraosseous extravascular pressure. This results in impaired venous drainage, which potentiates adipocyte edema and worsens the hypertension.

Table 2 General categorization of proposed underlying causes of avascular necrosis	
Categorization of Proposed Etiologies of Avascular Necrosis	
Vascular Disruption	Acute fractures, repetitive sporting activities, manual labor
Intravascular Obliteration	Fat emboli, sickle cell disease, systemic lupus erythematosus, antiphospholipid syndrome, factor V Leiden
Extraluminal Compression	Glucocorticoids increased adipocyte hypertrophy, compartment syndrome, Caisson disease, Gaucher disease

This effectively constitutes a "compartment syndrome of bone," and culminates in cellular ischemia and death. This initiates the above-outlined unbalanced process of reparative remodeling with net bone loss and results in the familiar fracture and collapse of Kienböck disease. They also point out that once fracture does occur, it will directly disrupt the subarticular venous plexus, which further contributes to intraosseous hypertension and potentiates this process.

Our pathophysiologic understanding of Kienböck disease informs our treatment algorithms. Surgical procedures have been designed to address each of the putative pathologic processes: vascular disruption, intravascular obliteration, and interosseous extravascular compression. Likely, due to the multifactorial cause, many of these procedures demonstrate varying degrees of success despite an imperfect understanding of the pathologic condition at play. Of course, once collapse occurs in later stages of disease, salvage procedures become the most appropriate surgical means of correction to include carpal replacement (**Fig. 4**), proximal row carpectomy, limited wrist arthrodesis, and total wrist arthrodesis.[61]

Earlier stages in disease may be treated with conservative management to include immobilization and anti-inflammatory medications for symptomatic relief (**Fig. 5**). However, these nonoperative management options may not ultimately change the progression of disease.

Vascular disruption

Obvious fracture or repetitive microtraumatic events initiate the process of AVN through vascular disruption. There can be considerable variation in lunate blood supply with roughly one-fifth of cadaveric models being at increased risk of AVN secondary to having a single palmar blood supply.[57,62,63] Once disrupted, neovascularization and angiogenesis seems limited and vascularized bone grafting serves as a viable treatment modality to prevent ongoing lunate collapse. There have been numerous vascularized bone-transfer procedures described[64,65]; however, the distal radius 4 + 5 extensor compartmental artery (4.5-ECA) bone graft is the most commonly used in the setting of Kienböck disease.[66] This graft provides a reasonable pedicle diameter with sufficient pedicle length and has shown favorable results. Moran and colleagues reviewed their outcomes in 26 patients undergoing 4,5-ECA bone grafting with supplemental fixation and showed the majority (71%) of lunates revascularized at long-term follow-up.[67] Ultimately, these revascularization procedures aim to correct the vascular disruption and provide viable osteoclasts and osteoblasts to allow for primary bone healing with accelerated creeping substitution.[68] As with all of these procedures, there is likely a mixed mechanism of action as the implantation of the bone flap also likely provides an effect similar to decompression in addressing extraluminal compression and addresses intravascular obliteration through direct bone replacement and neovascularization.

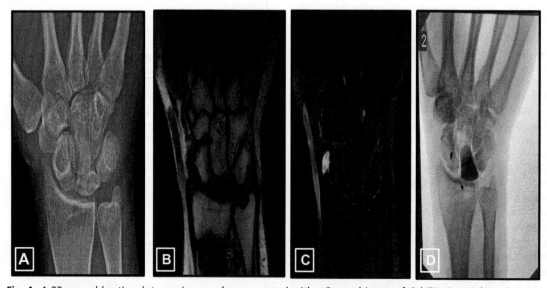

Fig. 4. A 23-year-old active duty service member presented with a 2-year history of debilitating right wrist pain. Their initial presenting images were concerning for subchondral collapse of their lunate (*A*) prompting further MRI evaluation. Low signal intensity on T1-weighted imaging (*B*) with increased signal intensity on T2-weighted imaging (*C*) was consistent with acute on chronic changes associated with advanced Kienböck disease. After failing conservative management, the patient elected to undergo a pyrocarbon lunate replacement (*D*).

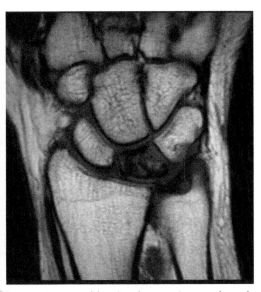

Fig. 5. A 31-year-old active duty service member who presented with insidious onset right wrist pain that progressed during a 3-month period. There were no visible changes on radiographic imaging. An MRI was ordered by their primary care provider for concern of ligamentous injury. The decreased signal intensity in their lunate on T1-weighted MRI coronal imaging without significant surrounding degenerative changes was consistent with early stage Kienböck disease. They were treated with a corticosteroid injection, nonsteroidal anti-inflammatory medications, and prolonged casting.

Extraluminal compression

Extraluminal compression thought to be addressed through the utilization of joint leveling procedures. These procedures mechanically unload the lunate through restoration of the distal radioulnar joint to a neutral or 1 mm ulnar-positive variance.[64] Ulnar-negative patients may be treated with ulnar lengthening; however, this is generally not recommended due to risk of nonunion, and as such, radial shortening osteotomies are often the procedure of choice for these patients[69–72] Ulnar-positive patients may be treated with radial closing wedge osteotomy, radial dome osteotomy, and most commonly with capitate shortening osteotomy.[69] These osteotomies attempt to increase the surface area between the radius and lunate so force transmission across the articulation is decreased. Joint leveling may decrease intraosseous pressure, decrease microtrauma, and shift load away from a bone with compromised internal trabecular structure.

Core decompression in the setting of early stage femoral head AVN has shown promising long-term results with cessation of disease progression.[73]

Lunate decompression is an analogous procedure aimed at decreasing the intraosseous pressure in early stage disease with similar results comparable to joint leveling procedures.[54] Direct comparison studies are needed to establish superiority between treatment modalities.

Intravascular obliteration

The focus of treatment in the setting of coagulopathy and sickle cell disease revolves around prevention. It can be assumed repeated vascular insults secondary to sickle cell crisis events increases the risk of AVN over time. For example, one series of sickle cell patients reported AVN in the femoral head of 11.1% of their cohort less than 21 years of age, whereas another series reported AVN in 37.2% of their patients older than 18 years of age.[74,75] Avoidance of sickling events with deterrence of low-oxygen tension environments may prove beneficial over time. Further, the likelihood of progression of disease in sickle cell patients is notably higher than expected in comparison to patients without sickle cell disease.[76] This may warrant earlier or even prophylactic procedures that would otherwise not be considered for earlier stages of disease. AVN secondary to hypercoagulable syndromes has been prophylactically treated with warfarin or enoxaparin[35]; however, proven efficacy is lacking.

Synopsis: Pathophysiology of Avascular Necrosis

Avascular necrosis is a complicated, multifactorial disease with a predisposition for certain anatomic locations to include the carpus. The cause of avascular necrosis is poorly understood; however, our current understanding groups the pathologic insult into 3 categories: (1) direct vascular disruption, (2) intravascular obliteration, or (3) extravascular compression for purposes of attribution of causation, prevention, and to provide a framework on which to design treatment. Prompt diagnosis in the earlier stages of disease may permit intervention to halt the progression. The low-incidence rate of carpal AVN poses a challenge in establishing adequately powered, control-based validated treatment options and therefore optimal surgical management remains a continued debate among hand surgeons with small case-series and expert opinion guiding most of our treatment decisions. There is significant opportunity for innovation and discovery in the field of avascular necrosis and are hopeful this article and many like it will continue to spur the next generation of researchers to continue to ask some of these unanswered questions.

CLINICS CARE POINTS

- Avascular necrosis of the carpus most commonly involves the lunate or the scaphoid, which have been coined as Kienböck disease and Preiser disease, respectively.
- There have been reported cases of vascular necrosis within all other carpal bones in following descending ordered rates of incidence: capitate, hamate, trapezium, trapezoid, triquetrum, and pisiform.
- Early stages of disease may not be appreciated on radiographic images. Patients with known risk factors should be considered for magnetic resonance imaging in order to aid in establishing the diagnosis.
- Although large validation studies are lacking, it is generally accepted that early stages of disease before cortical collapse can be treated with extended periods of immobilization.
- Later stages of disease with subsequent morphologic or arthritic changes to the wrist may be treated with continued conservative symptomatic treatment to include continued immobilization, lifestyle changes, corticosteroid injections, or a posterior interosseous neurectomy. More aggressive surgical options include vascularized bone grafts or salvage procedures such as proximal row carpectomy.
- It is important to discuss these treatment options with patients in order to ensure they make educated decisions regarding their care. Patients' lifestyles, activities of daily living and goals for treatment are paramount in determining the optimal conservative or surgical treatment options.

FINANCIAL DISCLOSURE

Each author certifies that he or she has no financial disclosures that might pose a conflict of interest in connection with the submitted article.

CONFLICT OF INTEREST

Each author certifies that he or she has no commercial associations (eg, consultancies, stock ownership, equity interest, patent/licensing arrangements, and so forth) that might pose a conflict of interest in connection with the submitted article.

DISCLOSURE

The views expressed in this publication are those of the author(s) and do not reflect the official policy or position of William Beaumont Army Medical Center, Department of the Army, Defense Health Agency, or the US Government.

REFERENCES

1. Amsallem L, Serane J, Zbili D, et al. Idiopathic bilateral lunate and triquetrum avascular necrosis: a case report. Hand Surg Rehabil 2016;35(5):367–70.
2. Botte MJ, Pacelli LL, Gelberman RH. Vascularity and osteonecrosis of the wrist. Orthop Clin North Am 2004;35(3):405–21, xi.
3. D'Agostino P, Townley WA, Roulot E. Bilateral avascular necrosis of the trapezoid. J Hand Surg Am 2011;36(10):1678–80.
4. De Smet L, Willemen D, Kimpe E, et al. Nontraumatic osteonecrosis of the capitate bone associated with gout. Ann Chir Main Memb Super 1993;12(3):210–2.
5. Garcia LA, Vaca JB. Avascular necrosis of the pisiform. J Hand Surg Br 2006;31(4):453–4.
6. García-López A, Cardoso Z, Ortega L. Avascular necrosis of trapezium bone: a case report. J Hand Surg Am 2002;27(4):704–6.
7. Herbert TJ, Lanzetta M. Idiopathic avascular necrosis of the scaphoid. J Hand Surg Br 1994;19(2):174–82.
8. Imam S, Aldridge C, Lyall H. Bilateral idiopathic avascular necrosis of the scaphoid: a rare case of Preiser's disease. J Bone Joint Surg Br 2009; 91(10):1400–2.
9. Kalainov DM, Cohen MS, Hendrix RW, et al. Preiser's disease: identification of two patterns. J Hand Surg Am 2003;28(5):767–78.
10. Lenoir H, Coulet B, Lazerges C, et al. Idiopathic avascular necrosis of the scaphoid: 10 new cases and a review of the literature. indications for Preiser's disease. Orthop Traumatol Surg Res 2012;98(4):390–7.
11. Lin JD, Strauch RJ. Preiser disease. J Hand Surg Am 2013;38(9):1833–4.
12. Manohara R, Sebastin SJ, Puhaindran ME. Post traumatic avascular necrosis of the proximal carpal row–a case report. Hand Surg 2015;20(3):466–70.
13. Match RM. Nonspecific avascular necrosis of the pisiform bone: a case report. J Hand Surg Am 1980;5(4):341–2.
14. Milliez PY, Kinh Kha H, Allieu Y, et al. [Idiopathic aseptic osteonecrosis of the capitate bone. Literature review apropos of 3 new cases]. Int Orthop 1991;15(2):85–94.
15. Peters SJ, Verstappen C, Degreef I, et al. Avascular necrosis of the hamate: three cases and review of the literature. J Wrist Surg 2014;3(4):269–74.
16. Peters SJ, Degreef I, De Smet L. Avascular necrosis of the capitate: report of six cases and review of the literature. J Hand Surg Eur Vol 2015;40(5):520–5.
17. Petsatodis E, Ditsios K, Konstantinou P, et al. A case of trapezium avascular necrosis treated conservatively. Case Rep Orthop 2017;2017:6936013.

18. Por YC, Chew WY, Tsou IY. Avascular necrosis of the triquetrum: a case report. Hand Surg 2005;10(1): 91–4.

19. Sturzenegger M, Mencarelli F. Avascular necrosis of the trapezoid bone. J Hand Surg Br 1998;23(4):550–1.

20. Zafra M, Carpintero P, Cansino D. Osteonecrosis of the trapezium treated with a vascularized distal radius bone graft. J Hand Surg Am 2004;29(6): 1098–101.

21. Wells ME, Nicholson TC, Macias RA, et al. Incidence of scaphoid fractures and associated injuries at US trauma centers. J Wrist Surg 2021;10(2):123–8.

22. Aaron RK, Dyke JP, Ciombor DM, et al. Perfusion abnormalities in subchondral bone associated with marrow edema, osteoarthritis, and avascular necrosis. Ann N Y Acad Sci 2007;1117:124–37.

23. Afshar A, Tabrizi A. Avascular necrosis of the carpal bones other than Kienböck Disease. J Hand Surg Am 2020;45(2):148–52.

24. Klement MR, Sharkey PF. The Significance of Osteoarthritis-associated Bone Marrow Lesions in the Knee. J Am Acad Orthop Surg 2019;27(20): 752–9.

25. Franceschi F, Franceschetti E, Paciotti M, et al. Surgical management of osteonecrosis of the humeral head: a systematic review. Knee Surg Sports Traumatol Arthrosc 2017;25(10):3270–8.

26. Harreld KL, Marker DR, Wiesler ER, et al. Osteonecrosis of the humeral head. J Am Acad Orthop Surg 2009;17(6):345–55.

27. Beaulé PE, Amstutz HC. Management of Ficat stage III and IV osteonecrosis of the hip. J Am Acad Orthop Surg 2004;12(2):96–105.

28. Lafforgue P. Pathophysiology and natural history of avascular necrosis of bone. Joint Bone Spine 2006;73(5):500–7.

29. Quintero JI, Van Royen K, Bouri F, et al. Avascular necrosis of the lunate secondary to perilunate fracture dislocation: case report and review of the literature. SAGE Open Med Case Rep 2021;9. 2050313X211032398.

30. THERKELSEN F, ANDERSEN K. Lunatomalacia. Acta Chir Scand 1949;97(6):503–26.

31. Stahl S, Stahl AS, Meisner C, et al. A systematic review of the etiopathogenesis of Kienböck's disease and a critical appraisal of its recognition as an occupational disease related to hand-arm vibration. BMC Musculoskelet Disord 2012;13:225.

32. Viegas SF, Wagner K, Patterson R, et al. Medial (hamate) facet of the lunate. J Hand Surg Am 1990;15(4):564–71.

33. Bain GI, Clitherow HD, Millar S, et al. The effect of lunate morphology on the 3-dimensional kinematics of the carpus. J Hand Surg Am 2015;40(1):81–9. e1.

34. Bain GI, MacLean SB, Yeo CJ, et al. The Etiology and Pathogenesis of Kienböck Disease. J Wrist Surg 2016;5(4):248–54.

35. Shah KN, Racine J, Jones LC, et al. Pathophysiology and risk factors for osteonecrosis. Curr Rev Musculoskelet Med 2015;8(3):201–9.

36. Jones JP. Fat embolism and osteonecrosis. Orthop Clin North Am 1985;16(4):595–633.

37. Huang TC, Li J, Moran SL. Bilateral Kienböck's disease in a child with Factor V Leiden thrombophilia: a case report. J Hand Surg Eur Vol 2019;44(8): 859–61.

38. Periasamy U, Chilutti M, Kaplan SL, et al. Prevalence of and associations with avascular necrosis after pediatric sepsis: a single-center retrospective study. Pediatr Crit Care Med 2022. https://doi.org/10. 1097/PCC.0000000000002880.

39. Angulo-Ardoy M, Ureña-Aguilera Á. Knee osteonecrosis after COVID-19. Fam Pract 2021;38(Suppl 1): i45–7.

40. Jones LC, Mont MA, Le TB, et al. Procoagulants and osteonecrosis. J Rheumatol 2003;30(4):783–91.

41. Zalavras C, Dailiana Z, Elisaf M, et al. Potential aetiological factors concerning the development of osteonecrosis of the femoral head. Eur J Clin Invest 2000;30(3):215–21.

42. Becker CG, Harpel PC. alpha2-Macroglobulin on human vascular endothelium. J Exp Med 1976; 144(1):1–9.

43. Cvirn G, Gallistl S, Koestenberger M, et al. Alpha 2-macroglobulin enhances prothrombin activation and thrombin potential by inhibiting the anticoagulant protein C/protein S system in cord and adult plasma. Thromb Res 2002;105(5):433–9.

44. Kerachian MA, Cournoyer D, Harvey EJ, et al. New insights into the pathogenesis of glucocorticoid-induced avascular necrosis: microarray analysis of gene expression in a rat model. Arthritis Res Ther 2010;12(3):R124.

45. Luan Y, Kong L, Howell DR, et al. Inhibition of ADAMTS-7 and ADAMTS-12 degradation of cartilage oligomeric matrix protein by alpha-2-macroglobulin. Osteoarthritis Cartilage 2008;16(11):1413–20.

46. Gavish H, Bab I, Tartakovsky A, et al. Human alpha 2-macroglobulin is an osteogenic growth peptide-binding protein. Biochemistry 1997;36(48):14883–8.

47. Zhang Y, Ge G, Greenspan DS. Inhibition of bone morphogenetic protein 1 by native and altered forms of alpha2-macroglobulin. J Biol Chem 2006;281(51): 39096–104.

48. Arlet J, Ficat P, Lartigue G, et al. [Clinical research on intraosseous pressure in the upper femoral metaphysis and epiphysis in humans. application to the diagnosis of ischemia and necrosis]. Rev Rhum Mal Osteoartic 1972;39(11):717–23.

49. Ficat RP. Idiopathic bone necrosis of the femoral head. early diagnosis and treatment. J Bone Joint Surg Br 1985;67(1):3–9.

50. Zizic TM, Lewis CG, Marcoux C, et al. The predictive value of hemodynamic studies in preclinical

ischemic necrosis of bone. J Rheumatol 1989;
16(12):1559–64.

51. Wang GJ, Dughman SS, Reger SI, et al. The effect of
core decompression on femoral head blood flow in
steroid-induced avascular necrosis of the femoral
head. J Bone Joint Surg Am 1985;67(1):121–4.

52. Wang GJ, Moga DB, Richemer WG, et al. Cortisone
induced bone changes and its response to lipid
clearing agents. Clin Orthop Relat Res 1978;130:
81–5.

53. Cui Q, Wang GJ, Su CC, et al. The Otto Aufranc
Award. Lovastatin prevents steroid induced adipo-
genesis and osteonecrosis. Clin Orthop Relat Res
1997;344:8–19.

54. Mehrpour SR, Kamrani RS, Aghamirsalim MR, et al.
Treatment of Kienböck disease by lunate core
decompression. J Hand Surg Am 2011;36(10):
1675–7.

55. Matsuo K, Hirohata T, Sugioka Y, et al. Influence of
alcohol intake, cigarette smoking, and occupational
status on idiopathic osteonecrosis of the femoral
head. Clin Orthop Relat Res 1988;234:115–23.

56. Large TM, Adams MR, Loeffler BJ, et al. Posttraumatic Avascular Necrosis After Proximal Femur,
Proximal Humerus, Talar Neck, and Scaphoid Fractures. J Am Acad Orthop Surg 2019;27(21):
794–805.

57. Panagis JS, Gelberman RH, Taleisnik J, et al. The
arterial anatomy of the human carpus. Part II: The intraosseous vascularity. J Hand Surg Am 1983;8(4):
375–82.

58. Glimcher MJ, Kenzora JE. Nicolas Andry award. The
biology of osteonecrosis of the human femoral head
and its clinical implications: 1. Tissue biology. Clin
Orthop Relat Res 1979;138:284–309.

59. Glimcher MJ, Kenzora JE. The biology of osteonecrosis of the human femoral head and its clinical implications: II. The pathological changes in the
femoral head as an organ and in the hip joint. Clin
Orthop Relat Res 1979;139:283–312.

60. Glimcher MJ, Kenzora JE. The biology of osteonecrosis of the human femoral head and its clinical implications. III. Discussion of the etiology and
genesis of the pathological sequelae; commments
on treatment. Clin Orthop Relat Res 1979;140:
273–312.

61. Rioux-Forker D, Shin AY. Osteonecrosis of the
lunate: Kienböck Disease. J Am Acad Orthop Surg
2020;28(14):570–84.

62. Freedman DM, Botte MJ, Gelberman RH. Vascularity of the carpus. Clin Orthop Relat Res 2001;
383:47–59.

63. Gelberman RH, Menon J. The vascularity of the
scaphoid bone. J Hand Surg Am 1980;5(5):508–13.

64. Lutsky K, Beredjiklian PK. Kienböck disease. J Hand
Surg Am 2012;37(9):1942–52.

65. Wells M, Klahs K, Polmear M, et al. Free-vascular-
ized bone grafts for scaphoid non-unions viable as
outpatient procedure? No 30-day complications in
NSQIP data. J Orthopaedic Business 2021;1(2):
5–8. Availble at. https://www.jorthobusiness.org/
index.php/jorthobusiness/article/view/6.

66. Elhassan BT, Shin AY. Vascularized bone grafting for
treatment of Kienböck's disease. J Hand Surg Am
2009;34(1):146–54.

67. Moran SL, Cooney WP, Berger RA, et al. The use of
the 4 + 5 extensor compartmental vascularized
bone graft for the treatment of Kienböck's disease.
J Hand Surg Am 2005;30(1):50–8.

68. Luo J, Diao E. Kienböck's disease: an approach to
treatment. Hand Clin 2006;22(4):465–73. ; abstract
vi.

69. Beredjiklian PK. Kienböck's disease. J Hand Surg
Am 2009;34(1):167–75.

70. Watanabe T, Takahara M, Tsuchida H, et al. Long-
term follow-up of radial shortening osteotomy for
Kienbock disease. J Bone Joint Surg Am 2008;
90(8):1705–11.

71. Raven EE, Haverkamp D, Marti RK. Outcome of
Kienböck's disease 22 years after distal radius
shortening osteotomy. Clin Orthop Relat Res 2007;
460:137–41.

72. Zenzai K, Shibata M, Endo N. Long-term outcome of
radial shortening with or without ulnar shortening for
treatment of Kienbock's disease: a 13-25 year
follow-up. J Hand Surg Br 2005;30(2):226–8.

73. Castro FP, Barrack RL. Core decompression and
conservative treatment for avascular necrosis of
the femoral head: a meta-analysis. Am J Orthop
(Belle Mead Nj) 2000;29(3):187–94.

74. Mukisi-Mukaza M, Elbaz A, Samuel-Leborgne Y,
et al. Prevalence, clinical features, and risk factors
of osteonecrosis of the femoral head among adults
with sickle cell disease. Orthopedics 2000;23(4):
357–63.

75. Matos MA, dos Santos Silva LL, Brito Fernandes R,
et al. Avascular necrosis of the femoral head in
sickle cell disease patients. Ortop Traumatol Rehabil
2012;14(2):155–60.

76. Hernigou P, Habibi A, Bachir D, et al. The natural history of asymptomatic osteonecrosis of the femoral
head in adults with sickle cell disease. J Bone Joint
Surg Am 2006;88(12):2565–72.

Vascular Supply of the Wrist

Courtney Carlson Strother, MD, Nicholas Pulos, MD*

KEYWORDS

- Vascular • Blood supply • Anatomy • Wrist • Carpus

KEY POINTS

- The scaphoid and capitate rely on a single vascular network in a retrograde fashion as the blood supply to most of the carpus.
- Most (80%) lunates are supplied by both a dorsal and volar vascular network, and approximately 20% of lunates have an isolated volar blood supply.
- Multiple volar and dorsal vascular arches across the wrist create a vast network of anastomoses from the radial, ulnar, and interosseous arteries.

INTRODUCTION

The vascularity of the wrist as previously described has been refined over time with advancement of imaging and dissection techniques. An understanding of this complex anatomy is vital in the understanding of many clinical processes such as scaphoid fracture nonunions and avascular necrosis of the lunate in Kienbock disease. Furthermore, multiple surgical techniques take advantage of the vascular network in the treatment of these disorders. This article reviews the blood supply of the distal radius, ulna, and carpal bones and its clinical implications.

DISTAL RADIUS AND ULNA VASCULAR ANATOMY
Dorsal Anatomy

The radial, ulnar, anterior interosseous, and posterior interosseous arteries are the 4 major vessels in the forearm that encompass the vascularity of the wrist. These arteries have multiple branches that form anastomoses, creating both volar and dorsal arches at the wrist. The dorsal distal radius and ulna are supplied by vessels named by their association with the extensor compartments of the wrist (**Fig. 1**A).[1] The 1,2 and 2,3 intercompartmental supraretinacular arteries (IC SRAs) lie between their named extensor compartments and are superficial to the retinaculum. The 1,2 IC SRA originates proximally in the forearm from the radial artery and forms an anastomosis distally with the radial artery, radiocarpal arch, and/or the intercarpal arch. Nutrient vessels from the 1,2 IC SRA penetrate the retinaculum to provide blood supply to the distal radius. The 2,3 IC SRA most commonly originates proximally from the anterior interosseous artery or the posterior division of the anterior interosseous artery and joins the dorsal intercarpal arch, the dorsal radiocarpal arch, and/or the fourth extensor compartment artery distally. This vessel lies on the dorsal radial tubercle (Lister tubercle) and provides nutrient vessels into the distal radius.[1]

The fourth and fifth extensor compartment arteries lie within their respective extensor compartments or within the retinaculum septae. The fourth extensor compartment artery often rests next to the posterior interosseous nerve and most commonly forms an anastomosis with the dorsal intercarpal arch.[1] The fifth extensor compartment artery is the largest of the dorsal extensor arteries and joins distally with the dorsal intercarpal arch. Nutrient vessels from the fourth and fifth extensor compartment arteries provide blood supply to the ulnar border of the distal radius.[1] In addition, 1 to 3 oblique dorsal arteries supply the distal ulna, often

Department of Orthopaedic Surgery, Mayo Clinic, 200 1st Street Southwest, Rochester, MN 55905, USA
* Corresponding author.
E-mail address: pulos.nicholas@mayo.edu

Hand Clin 38 (2022) 377–384
https://doi.org/10.1016/j.hcl.2022.03.001

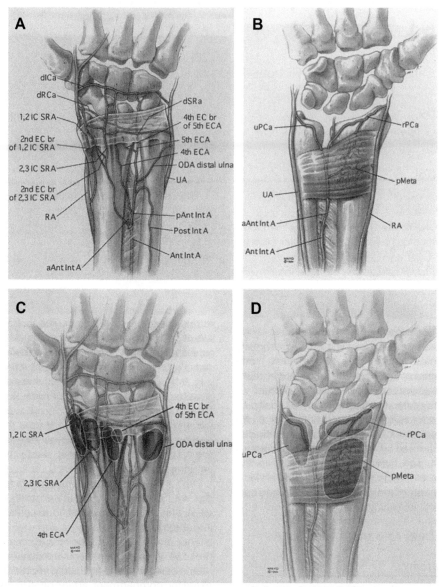

Fig. 1. (*A*) Dorsal and (*B*) palmar distal radius and ulna showing extraosseous vessels. (*C*) Dorsal and (*D*) palmar distal radius and ulna with shaded regions showing where nutrient vessels from the labeled arteries penetrate bone. aAnt Int A, anterior division of the anterior interosseous artery; Ant Int A, anterior interosseous artery; dICa, dorsal intercarpal arch; dRCa, dorsal radiocarpal arch; dSRa, dorsal supraretinacular arch; 2nd EC br of 1,2 IC SRA, second extensor compartment branch of 1,2 intercompartmental supraretinacular artery; 4th ECA, fourth extensor compartment artery; 5th ECA, fifth extensor compartment artery; 4th EC br of 5th ECA, fourth extensor compartment branch of fifth extensor compartment artery; 1,2 IC SRA, 1,2 intercompartmental supraretinacular artery; 2,3 IC SRA, 2,3 intercompartmental supraretinacular artery; ODA distal ulna, oblique dorsal artery of the distal ulna; pAnt Int A, posterior division of the anterior interosseous artery; pMeta, palmar metaphyseal arch; Post Int A, posterior interosseous artery; RA, radial artery; rPCa, radial half of palmar carpal arch; UA, ulnar artery; uPCa, ulnar half of palmar carpal arch. (*From* Sheetz KK, Bishop AT, Berger RA. The arterial blood supply of the distal radius and ulna and its potential use in vascularized pedicled bone grafts. J Hand Surg Am. 1995;20(6):902-914.; with permission)

arising from an arch between the anterior and posterior interosseous arteries.[1]

The dorsal wrist contains 4 described arches that connect many of the previously mentioned

arteries (**Fig. 2**).[1–3] The dorsal radiocarpal arch runs deep to the extensor tendons and is supplied by the radial and ulnar arteries and additional vessels, such as the 1,2 IC SRA, the 2,3 IC SRA, and/

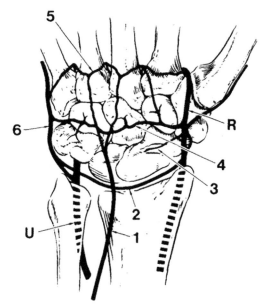

Fig. 2. The arterial supply of the dorsum of the wrist. U, ulnar artery; 1, dorsal branch of the anterior interosseous artery; 2, dorsal radiocarpal arch; 3, branch to the dorsal ridge of the scaphoid; 4, dorsal intercarpal arch; 5, basal metacarpal arch; 6, medial branch of the ulnar artery. (*From* Gelberman RH, Panagis JS, Taleisnik J, Baumgaertner M. The arterial anatomy of the human carpus. Part I: The extraosseous vascularity. J Hand Surg Am. 1983;8(4):367-375.; with permission)

or the fourth and fifth extensor compartment arteries.[1] The dorsal radiocarpal arch provides blood supply to the far distal end of the distal radius through small nutrient arteries.[1] In addition, the nutrient vessels from this arch supply the lunate and triquetrum.[2] The dorsal intercarpal arch is formed from the radial, ulnar, and fifth extensor compartment arteries and is the largest of the dorsal arches.[1,2] This arch runs between the proximal and distal carpal rows. The dorsal intercarpal arch anastomoses with the radiocarpal arch, and both contribute to the blood supply of the lunate and triquetrum.[2]

Two additional dorsal arches at the wrist are the basal metacarpal transverse arch and the dorsal supraretinacular arch.[1,2] These arches are less pronounced and often described as a network of anastomosing vessels. The basal metacarpal transverse arch is supplied by deep perforating branches from the deep palmar arch and is incomplete in most patients.[2] This arch forms anastomoses with the intercarpal arch to supply the distal carpal row.[2] The dorsal supraretinacular arch connects the dorsal extensor arteries and originates from the 1,2 IC SRA, connecting to the ulnar artery through a series of vessels.[1]

Pedicled vascularized bone grafts have been described using the 1,2 IC SRA[1,4] and 2,3 IC SRA[1] for treatment of carpal avascular necrosis, nonunions, or as bone graft for arthrodesis (**Fig. 1**C). In addition, Sheetz and colleagues[1] described the fourth extensor compartment artery pedicled vascularized bone graft, and they found these pedicles could be lengthened using the fifth extensor compartment artery as a large retrograde conduit to the fourth extensor compartment artery, 1,2 IC SRA, or 2,3 IC SRA.

Volar Anatomy

The palmar blood supply of the wrist is composed of additional transverse arches stemming from the radial, ulnar, and anterior interosseous arteries (**Fig. 1**B, **Fig. 3**).[1,2] Most proximally, the palmar metaphyseal arch runs through the pronator quadratus muscle and provides blood supply to the radial metaphysis.[1] At the radiocarpal and ulnocarpal joints, the palmar carpal[1] or palmar radiocarpal arch[2] supplies the extreme distal aspects of the radius and ulna. The anterior interosseous artery bifurcates this arch into radial and ulnar halves that anastomose with the radial and ulnar arteries, respectively.[1] In addition, a palmar intercarpal arch has been described between the proximal and distal carpal rows, although this was present in approximately half of the studied specimens.[2] Most distally, the deep palmar arch supplies the trapezoid, capitate, and hamate through recurrent arteries.[2] The palmar carpal arch has been described as a pedicled vascularized muscle-bone graft using the pronator quadratus (**Fig. 1**D), although this graft has less reliable vascularity and a short pedicle length, limiting its use.[1,5–8]

CARPAL VASCULAR ANATOMY
Scaphoid

The blood supply to the carpal bones have been extensively explored over the last century, particularly the scaphoid and lunate in the clinical setting of avascular necrosis. The scaphoid is the most commonly fractured carpal bone, with a high incidence of avascular necrosis in the proximal pole.[9,10] The radial artery supplies most of the blood to the scaphoid; however, dorsal and volar branches of the anterior interosseous artery provide collateral vascularity through anastomoses with the dorsal and volar radial artery branches, respectively.[11] Dorsal radial vessels penetrate the dorsal scaphoid ridge and travel in a retrograde fashion to supply the proximal 70% to 83% of the scaphoid.[11,12] The distal 17% to 30% of the scaphoid is supplied through the tubercle

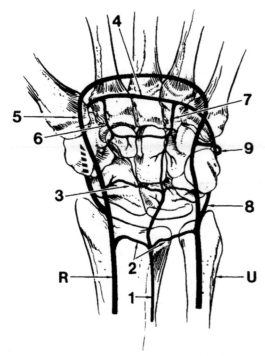

Fig. 3. The arterial supply of the palmar aspect of the wrist. 1, palmar branch of the anterior interosseous artery; 2, palmar radiocarpal arch; 3, palmar intercarpal arch; 4, deep palmar arch; 5, superficial palmar arch; 6, radial recurrent artery; 7, ulnar recurrent artery; 8, medial branch of the ulnar artery; 9, branch off ulnar artery contributing to the dorsal intercarpal arch. (*From* Gelberman RH, Panagis JS, Taleisnik J, Baumgaertner M. The arterial anatomy of the human carpus. Part I: The extraosseous vascularity. J Hand Surg Am. 1983;8(4):367-375.; with permission)

from the superficial palmar branch or direct volar radial artery branches.[11,12] The cross-sectional area of the dorsal vessels to the scaphoid were more than double that of the volar vessels.[12] Supplemental volar waist vessels were discovered in 4 of 13 (31%) specimens in a study by Morsy and colleagues[12] In addition, these investigators found rare interosseous anastomosing vessels in 2 of 13 specimens, where Gelberman and Menon found no evidence of interosseous anastomoses.[11] Given the dominant dorsal blood supply to the scaphoid, Gelberman and Menon[11] recommended a volar operative approach to the scaphoid as a lesser insult to the scaphoid blood supply.

Using microcomputed tomography (micro-CT), Morsy and colleagues[12] described 2 types of scaphoids and their significance to their vascularity. Type I, or full scaphoids, had a significantly higher number of vascular branches supplying most of the scaphoid than type II, or slender, scaphoids (**Fig. 4**). They suggested some

scaphoids, particularly type II scaphoids, are at higher risk of developing avascular necrosis. Furthermore, they recommended placing scaphoid screws across the central or antegrade axis of the scaphoid to have the lowest disruptive effect on interosseous blood supply.[12]

Lunate

The lunate is the second most common carpal bone to undergo avascular necrosis and was first described by Kienbock in the early 1900s. Most lunates receive blood supply from both dorsal and volar vessels.[13–17] Dorsally, the intercarpal branch from the radial artery is the largest supply to the lunate,[17] with additional contributions noted from a branch at the level of the radiocarpal arch and a branch from the anterior interosseous artery. Volarly, the ulnar, radial, volar anterior interosseous artery, and recurrent branch off the deep palmar arch all contribute to a vascular plexus the supplies the volar lunate.[17] Using micro-CT technology, an average of 1.4 and 2.3 vessels were found entering the dorsal and volar lunate, respectively.[16] The difference in vessel number was found to be statistically significant, but the diameters of the vessels were not significantly different between the volar and dorsal arteries.[16] A comparison of the internal vascularity found no significant difference in contributions between the volar and dorsal blood supply to the lunate[16]; however, 14.3%[16] to 20%[15] of lunates studied were found to have no dorsal blood supply to the lunate. A dorsal surgical approach to the lunate is therefore recommended to protect the more consistent volar blood supply.[16]

The internal lunate vascularity was described by Gelberman and colleagues[17] as forming 3 main vascular patterns: Y, I, and X. Y-shaped lunate vascularity is the most common pattern, followed by I, then X.[16] These patterns are formed by the volar and dorsal vessels forming anastomoses at the midportion of the lunate, typically just distal to the center of the bone.[17] The long axis of the lunate has the highest vascularity, and the proximal pole of the lunate is relatively avascular.[16,17] No difference in vascularity was found between type I and II lunates.[16] Given the interosseous vascular patterns of the lunate, van Alphen and colleagues[16] proposed a safe zone for surgical drills, screws, and anchor placement on the dorsal, radial half of the lunate (**Fig. 5**).

Capitate

The capitate is another carpal bone that receives its blood supply predominantly in a retrograde fashion.[15,18] Both volar and dorsal vessels enter

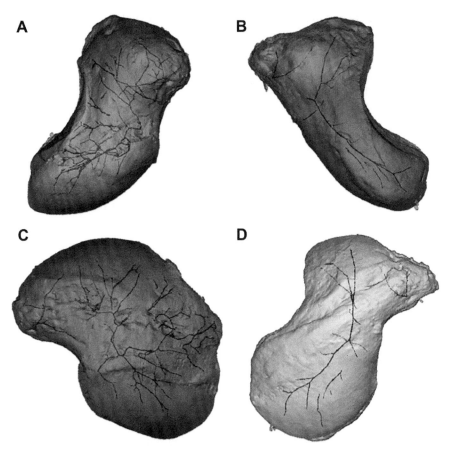

Fig. 4. Comparison between the internal vascularity of (*A* and *C*) type I and (*B* and *D*) type II scaphoids. (*From* Morsy M, Sabbagh MD, van Alphen NA, Laungani AT, Kadar A, Moran SL. The Vascular Anatomy of the Scaphoid: New Discoveries Using Micro-Computed Tomography Imaging. J Hand Surg Am. 2019;44(11):928-938.; with permission)

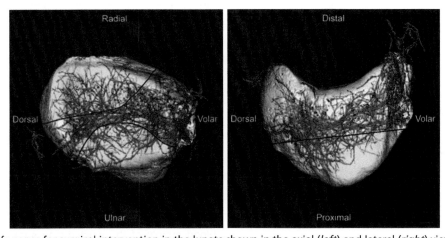

Fig. 5. Safe zones for surgical intervention in the lunate shown in the axial (*left*) and lateral (*right*) views (*yellow shaded areas*). These zones correspond to the areas of less vasculature. (*From* van Alphen NA, Morsy M, Laungani AT, et al. A Three-Dimensional Micro-Computed Tomographic Study of the Intraosseous Lunate Vasculature: Implications for Surgical Intervention and the Development of Avascular Necrosis. Plast Reconstr Surg. 2016;138(5):869e-878e; with permission)

the distal half of the capitate and form anastomoses in approximately 30% of patients.[15,18] Panagis and colleagues[15] reported a predominance of the dorsal supply in their cadaveric study, although a more recent evaluation of the capitate vascularity by micro-CT found no difference between volar and dorsal vascular systems.[15,18] Additional vessels entering the proximal pole of the capitate through the volar capitate ligaments were found in up to 70% of studied wrists.[18] These proximal pole vessels are postulated to explain the rarity of proximal pole avascular necrosis of the capitate following fractures, despite the largely retrograde blood supply.[18]

Trapezium

The vascularity of the trapezium stems from the radial artery and involves dorsal, volar, and lateral vessels entering into the respective nonarticular surfaces of the bone.[15,19] These vessels form both extraosseous and interosseous anastomoses, creating a rich arterial network around the carpus.[15,19] The dorsoradial aspect of the trapezium contains the predominant blood supply in most cases, and a cadaveric study by Goubau and colleagues[19] advocated a volar approach to the trapezium for surgical osteotomies to preserve this blood supply.[15,19]

Trapezoid

Similar to the trapezium, the dorsal blood supply is the predominant vascularity of trapezoid. One to 2 small volar vessels provide additional vascularity, but no anastomoses have been described between the dorsal and volar vessels interosseously.[15]

Hamate

The major blood supply to the hamate consists of 1 artery that enters the bone at the base of the hook of hamate.[15] This vessel often forms interosseous anastomosis with a network of dorsal nutrient vessels to the body of the hamate, but rare anastomoses from these vessels reach the hook of the hamate. Instead, the hook is often supplied by 1 or 2 small arteries that enter at the base or tip of the hook.[15,20] This vascular network to the hook is thought to contribute to the increased risk of hamate hook nonunions and avascular necrosis.[20]

Triquetrum

The triquetrum is an additional carpal bone that receives most of its blood supply through dorsal nutrient vessels penetrating nonarticular surfaces of the bone. Volarly, nutrient vessels proximal and distal to the pisiform facet provide additional supply, and most triquetrums have rich networks of interosseous anastomoses between this volar and dorsal vascularity.[15]

Pisiform

The pisiform has a vast vascular network that forms an arterial ring within the bone. Proximal and distal nutrient vessels within the tendon of the flexor carpi ulnaris provide equal blood supply to the pisiform, and no aspects of the bone are considered to be at risk of developing avascular necrosis.[15]

DISCUSSION

Our understanding of the vascularity of the wrist has a multitude of clinical implications and has been postulated as a cause of carpal disorders such as avascular necrosis and fracture nonunions. Gelberman classified the carpal bones into 3 groups based on their blood supply and risk of developing avascular necrosis (Table 1).[15,21] Group I is at the highest risk of developing avascular necrosis because of a large portion of the bone relying on 1 area of blood supply, and this group includes the scaphoid, capitate, and lunates with only volar blood supply. However, the finding of small vessels penetrating the proximal pole of the capitate may explain the lower rate of avascular necrosis in the capitate compared with the lunate and scaphoid.[18] Group II is considered to have moderate risk of developing avascular necrosis because of a lack of interosseous anastomoses between at least 2 sources of blood supply to the bone.[15] The hamate and trapezoid are included in group II, and hook of hamate fracture nonunions are considered to occur in part because of the poor blood supply to the hook.[20,22] Last, group III carpal bones have multiple sources of blood supply and a rich network of interosseous anastomoses.[15] These are considered to be at the lowest risk of developing avascular necrosis and include the trapezium, triquetrum, pisiform, and lunates with both dorsal and volar blood supply.[15]

In addition to identifying bones at risk for developing avascular necrosis, studies on vascular anatomy of the wrist have provided recommendations to decrease the risk of iatrogenic injury to the blood supply of the wrist during surgery. These considerations include a volar open approach to the scaphoid,[11] placing screws through the central or antegrade axis of the scaphoid,[12] a dorsal surgical approach to the lunate,[17] and instrumenting

Table 1
Blood supply to the carpus

Carpal Bone	Group[a]	Vessel Entry	Dominant Blood Supply	Interosseous Connections
Scaphoid	I	Volar, dorsal, volar	Dorsal	None
Capitate	I	Dorsal, capitate neck	Dorsal	Rare
Lunate (20%)	I	Volar, volar	Volar	None
Hamate	II	Dorsal, medial hook	Volar	Yes, no anastomoses between body and hook
Trapezoid	II	Volar, dorsal	Dorsal	None
Trapezium	III	Dorsal, lateral	Dorsal	Yes
Triquetrum	III	Volar, Dorsal	Dorsal	Yes
Pisiform	III	Proximal, Distal	Equal	Yes
Lunate (80%)	III	Volar, Dorsal	Volar	Yes: Y, X, and I patterns

[a] Groups classified by Panagis et al.[15]

the lunate on the dorsoradial aspect of the carpus if able.[16]

In addition, the intricate arches of the volar and dorsal wrist can be used to create vascularized bone grafts. These pedicled vascularized bone grafts are thought to improve healing in the setting of nonunion and/or avascular necrosis, and they are often used in treatment of scaphoid fracture nonunions with proximal pole necrosis or lunate avascular necrosis.[1,4,6–8,23–25]

SUMMARY

Understanding of the vascular anatomy to the wrist is not only important in understanding the cause of various carpal disorders but is imperative in avoiding iatrogenic injury to the carpal blood supply. Furthermore, surgeons can take advantage of this blood supply by keeping pedicled vascular bone grafts in their armamentarium for the treatment of carpal avascular necrosis or fracture nonunions.

CLINICS CARE POINTS

- Branches of the radial, ulnar, and interosseous arteries form multiple dorsal and volar vascular arches at the wrist.

- The scaphoid, capitate, and 20% of lunates with an isolated volar blood supply are at higher risk of developing avascular necrosis because of a large portion of the bone relying on a single blood supply.

- The trapezium, triquetrum, pisiform, and 80% of lunates with dorsal and volar vascularity are supplied by multiple nutrient vessels that form interosseous anastomoses thought to be protective of avascular necrosis.

- Dorsal approaches to the scaphoid, volar approaches to the lunate, and instrumentation of the lunate through the volar or ulnar half of the dorsal surface may place the scaphoid and lunate at increased risk of iatrogenic avascular necrosis.

- The 1,2 IC SRA, 2,3 IC SRA, fourth extensor compartment artery, and the fifth extensor compartment artery are dorsally based pedicled vascularized bone grafts that can be used in the treatment of carpal avascular necrosis, fracture nonunion, or in the setting of arthrodesis.

DISCLOSURE

The authors have nothing to disclose.

REFERENCES

1. Sheetz KK, Bishop AT, Berger RA. The arterial blood supply of the distal radius and ulna and its potential use in vascularized pedicled bone grafts. J Hand Surg Am 1995;20(6):902–14.
2. Gelberman RH, Panagis JS, Taleisnik J, et al. The arterial anatomy of the human carpus. Part I: The extraosseous vascularity. J Hand Surg Am 1983;8(4):367–75.
3. Freedman DM, Botte MJ, Gelberman RH. Vascularity of the carpus. Clin Orthop Relat Res 2001;383:47–59.
4. Zaidemberg C, Siebert JW, Angrigiani C. A new vascularized bone graft for scaphoid nonunion. J Hand Surg Am 1991;16(3):474–8.
5. Fontaine C, Millot F, Blancke D, et al. Anatomic basis of pronator quadratus flap. Surg Radiol Anat 1992;14(4):295–9.
6. Kuhlmann JN, Mimoun M, Boabighi A, et al. Vascularized bone graft pedicled on the volar carpal artery for non-union of the scaphoid. J Hand Surg Br 1987;12(2):203–10.

7. Leung PC, Hung LK. Use of pronator quadratus bone flap in bony reconstruction around the wrist. J Hand Surg Am 1990;15(4):637–40.

8. Rath S, Hung LK, Leung PC. Vascular anatomy of the pronator quadratus muscle-bone flap: a justification for its use with a distally based blood supply. J Hand Surg Am 1990;15(4):630–6.

9. Hove LM. Epidemiology of scaphoid fractures in Bergen, Norway. Scand J Plast Reconstr Surg Hand Surg 1999;33(4):423–6.

10. Leslie IJ, Dickson RA. The fractured carpal scaphoid. Natural history and factors influencing outcome. J Bone Joint Surg Br 1981;63-b(2):225–30.

11. Gelberman RH, Menon J. The vascularity of the scaphoid bone. J Hand Surg Am 1980;5(5):508–13.

12. Morsy M, Sabbagh MD, van Alphen NA, et al. The vascular anatomy of the scaphoid: new discoveries using micro-computed tomography imaging. J Hand Surg Am 2019;44(11):928–38.

13. Dubey PP, Chauhan NK, Siddiqui MS, et al. Study of vascular supply of lunate and consideration applied to Kienböck disease. Hand Surg 2011;16(1):9–13.

14. Lamas C, Carrera A, Proubasta I, et al. The anatomy and vascularity of the lunate: considerations applied to Kienböck's disease. Chir Main 2007;26(1):13–20.

15. Panagis JS, Gelberman RH, Taleisnik J, et al. The arterial anatomy of the human carpus. Part II: The intraosseous vascularity. J Hand Surg Am 1983;8(4):375–82.

16. van Alphen NA, Morsy M, Laungani AT, et al. A three-dimensional micro-computed tomographic study of the intraosseous lunate vasculature: implications for surgical intervention and the development of avascular necrosis. Plast Reconstr Surg 2016;138(5):869e–78e.

17. Gelberman RH, Bauman TD, Menon J, et al. The vascularity of the lunate bone and Kienböck's disease. J Hand Surg Am 1980;5(3):272–8.

18. Kadar A, Morsy M, Sur YJ, et al. The vascular anatomy of the capitate: new discoveries using micro-computed tomography imaging. J Hand Surg Am 2017;42(2):78–86.

19. Goubau JF, Benis S, Van Hoonacker P, et al. Vascularization of the trapeziometacarpal joint and its clinical importance: anatomical study. Chir Main 2012;31(2):57–61.

20. Failla JM. Hook of hamate vascularity: vulnerability to osteonecrosis and nonunion. J Hand Surg Am 1993;18(6):1075–9.

21. Gelberman RH, Gross MS. The vascularity of the wrist. Identification of arterial patterns at risk. Clin Orthop Relat Res 1986;(202):40–9.

22. Kadar A, Bishop AT, Suchyta MA, et al. Diagnosis and management of hook of hamate fractures. J Hand Surg Eur 2018;43(5):539–45.

23. Moran SL, Cooney WP, Berger RA, et al. The use of the 4 + 5 extensor compartmental vascularized bone graft for the treatment of Kienböck's disease. J Hand Surg Am 2005;30(1):50–8.

24. Mouilhade F, Auquit-Auckbur I, Duparc F, et al. Anatomical comparative study of two vascularized bone grafts for the wrist. Surg Radiol Anat 2007;29(1):15–20.

25. Oppikofer C, Büchler U, Schmid E. The surgical anatomy of the dorsal carpal branch of the ulnar artery: basis for a neurovascular dorso-ulnar pedicled flap. Surg Radiol Anat 1992;14(2):97–101.

Kienböck Disease
Clinical Presentation, Epidemiology, and Historical Perspective

Charles Andrew Daly, MD[a],*, Alexander Reed Graf, MD[b],*

KEYWORDS

- Lunate avascular necrosis • Kienböck disease • Epidemiology • Carpal collapse • Carpal instability
- Wrist arthritis

KEY POINTS

- Kienböck disease is a rare osteonecrosis of the lunate secondary to mechanical and biological factors
- Kienböck disease most commonly affects men aged 20 to 40 years with a variable clinical presentation
- Kienböck disease can lead to lunate collapse, carpal instability, and arthritis
- Advanced imaging, as well as wrist arthroscopy, can be helpful for accurate staging and selecting the appropriate treatment

HISTORICAL PERSPECTIVE

Throughout history, technological innovation has served as a catalyst for scientific discovery. Before the development of x-rays by German physicist Wilhelm Roentgen in 1895, early anatomists relied on cadaveric dissection to understand carpal anatomy and pathology. These early dissections revealed several congenital lunate abnormalities, such as lunatum partitum, bipartitum, hypolunatum, and epilunatum.[1] Later, the French physician Peste was the first to describe lunate collapse on an autopsy specimen from a patient who fell from height in 1843.[1]

Lunate collapse secondary to osteonecrosis was first described in a living patient in 1910. Robert Kienböck, an Austrian pioneer in the field of radiology, was the first to describe the clinical and radiographic changes of lunate osteonecrosis in the disease that now bears his name in 16 of his own patients[2–4] (**Fig. 1**). In his series, patients were largely male laborers presenting with wrist pain in

their third and fourth decade of life. At the time, he postulated that the changes to lunate structure and shape could be secondary to congenital anomaly, compression fracture, infection, or inflammatory arthritis; however, he ultimately favored "a disturbance in the nutrition of the lunate caused by rupture of the ligaments and blood vessels during contusions, sprains, or subluxations" to be the root cause of what he called "lunatomalacia."[5]

The belief that a subtle traumatic event that resulted in a vascular insult to the lunate was responsible for subsequent osteonecrosis, carpal collapse, and arthritis prevailed over the next several decades. In 1925, Goldsmith was the first to describe an idiopathic lunate fracture without preceding trauma in the American literature.[3] He agreed with Kienböck in believing that lunate subluxation with spontaneous reduction was responsible for disruption to the dorsal ligaments and, therefore, lunate nutritional supply.[1] In his case series of 3 patients, he described 4 clinical stages of

a Department of Orthopaedic Surgery, Division of Upper Extremity Surgery, Medical University of South Carolina, Medical University of South Carolina Orthopaedics, 96 Jonathan Lucas Street, MSC Code: 708, Charleston, SC 29425, USA; b Department of Orthopedic Surgery, Division of Upper Extremity Surgery, Emory University, Emory Orthopaedics & Spine Center, 21 Ortho Lane, Atlanta, GA 30329, USA
* Corresponding authors.
E-mail addresses: dalyc@musc.edu (C.A.D.); Alexander.reed.graf@emory.edu (A.R.G.)

Hand Clin 38 (2022) 385–392
https://doi.org/10.1016/j.hcl.2022.03.002
0749-0712/22/© 2022 Elsevier Inc. All rights reserved.

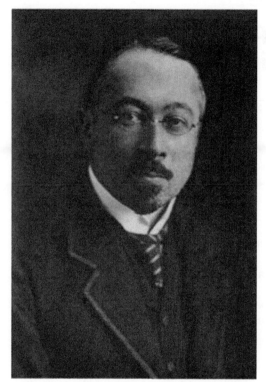

Fig. 1. Robert Kienböck (1871–1953). (*From* Chochole M. Robert Kienbock: the man and his work. J Hand Surg Eur Vol. 2010;35(7):534-537. https://doi.org/10. 1177/1753193410367708; with permission.)

Kienböck disease: (1) joint irritation stage following trauma, (2) an asymptomatic stage, (3) a symptomatic disease stage, and (4) a stage of moderate disability.[6]

In 1928, Hultén was the first to describe the normal distribution of ulnar wrist variance in the Swedish population as well as identify a significant correlation between ulnar negative variance and development of Kienböck disease.[7] In his radiographic analysis of 400 wrists, he found that ulnar variance was distributed in a bell shape curve, with most individuals being ulnar neutral (61%), followed by ulnar negative (23%) and ulnar positive (16%).[1] In addition, subsequent analysis of 23 patients with Kienböck disease in his series revealed 17 (74%) with ulnar negative wrists and 6 (26%) to have ulnar neutral wrists, with no patients with Kienböck disease having ulnar positive variance.

This anatomic observation that ulnar negative variance was associated with the development of Kienböck disease led to the development of joint leveling procedures to redistribute forces across the lunate and limit the progression of disease. In 1945, Persson reported his series of 19 corrective osteotomies (3 radial shortening and 16 ulnar lengthening) for treatment of Kienböck disease in

patients with ulnar negative variance.[1,8] However, results from these initial efforts were limited by contemporary methods of fixation, which consisted of only cerclage wires at the time. Nonetheless, he observed a 50% improvement in lunate structure following his corrective osteotomy.[1]

Kienböck belief that a dorsal ligamentous injury led to disruption in the vascular supply to the lunate was later challenged by Stahl in 1947.[9] Through study of arteriograms of the wrist, he found the volar circulation to be the dominant blood supply to be lunate and postulated that injury to these small vessels may be the inciting pathology of Kienböck disease.[1] He also was the first to propose a radiographic staging system for Kienböck disease, which endured until subsequent revision by Lichtman 30 years later (**Table 1**).[10,11] In Stahl's original staging system, Kienböck disease began as a radiodense lunate fracture (stage 1), followed by secondary bony resorption with development of a rarefaction line (stage 2), diffuse lunate sclerosis (stage 3), then secondary fractures with fragmentation (stage 4), and then ultimately arthrosis (stage 5).[1] Lichtman's revised classification system added details provided by computed tomography (CT) and MRI, demonstrating disease progression from lunate edema to sclerosis, fracture, and collapse, followed by carpal instability and arthritis (**Fig. 2**).[11,12]

The controversy surrounding the dominant blood supply to the lunate was resolved in 1980 when Gelberman published his cadaveric study detailing the extensive intraosseous and extraosseous lunate vascular anatomy.[13] In 35 cadavers, the radial and ulnar arteries were injected with Ward's blue latex and subsequently processed and sectioned. Gelberman found the extraosseous vascular supply was constituted by a system of 2 to 3 dorsal vessels and 3 to 4 volar vessels feeding carpal vascular plexuses over the dorsal and volar poles of the lunate.[13] These nutrient vessels were also found to enter the lunate through distinct foramina.[13,14] The intraosseous vascular supply was described in 3 patterns based on these perforating nutrient vessels: "Y" (59%), "X" (31%), and "I" (10%), with the "I" pattern being most susceptible to injury due to only having one nutrient vessel from each side of the lunate.[13]

In 1993, Jensen confirmed decreased vascularity of the lunate in patients with Kienböck disease using technetium 99m-methylene diphosphonate scintigraphy.[15] However, in his case series of 10 patients, he was also able to measure intraosseous lunate pressure using a 14-gauge needle with a transducer and compared the values to the adjacent capitate and radial styloid pressure measurements.[15] He found that in

Table 1
Lichtman classification for Kienböck disease (1977)

Stage	Imaging Findings
I	Normal on XR and CT; increased bone edema on MRI
II	Sclerosis present on XR; no collapse; MRI with low T1 signal intensity, variable T2 intensity
IIIA	Lunate collapse present; radioscaphoid angle < 60°
IIIB	Lunate collapse present; radioscaphoid angle > 60° (fixed)
IV	Radiocarpal and/or midcarpal arthritis present

patients with Kienböck disease, the lunate pressures were significantly higher than in the capitate and radial styloid pressures. He concluded that the avascular changes must be due to a lack of venous outflow relative to arterial inflow similar to avascular necrosis elsewhere in the body.[15]

Although the precise etiology of Kienböck disease remains unknown, it is now believed that predisposing factors such as vascular insufficiency, elevated intraosseous pressure, repetitive lunate microtrauma, and anatomic factors (such as negative ulnar variance, increased uncovering of the lunate, abnormal radial inclination, and a trapezoidal lunate shape) all play a role in the development of Kienböck disease.[14,15]

EPIDEMIOLOGY

The true prevalence of Kienböck disease is not entirely known as the early stages of disease are often asymptomatic and the timing of disease progression is highly variable. However, Kienböck disease is considered a "rare disease" by the Office of Rare Diseases (ORD) of the National Institutes of Health (NIH), and it currently affects less than 200,000 people in the United States.[16–18]

Previous studies have estimated the asymptomatic prevalence to be between 1% and 2% in African and Japanese populations, respectively.[15,16] Recently, a large retrospective analysis of over 51,000 American patients who received wrist

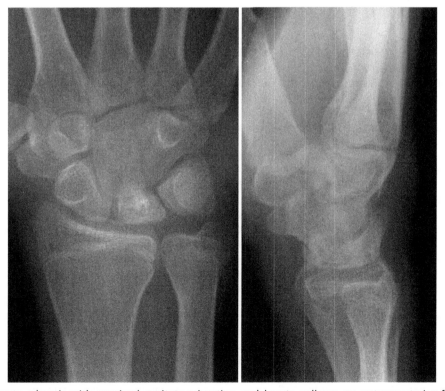

Fig. 2. Lunate sclerosis with proximal capitate migration and lunate collapse on anteroposterior film (left). Lateral film reveals radioscaphoid angle less than 60°, consistent with Lichtman IIIA (right). (*From* Jafarnia K, Collins ED, Kohl HW 3rd, Bennett JB, Ilahi OA. Reliability of the Lichtman classification of Kienböck's disease. J Hand Surg Am. 2000;25(3):529-534. https://doi.org/10.1053/jhsu.2000.7377; with permission.)

radiographs for other reasons than suspected Kienböck disease found an overall incidence of Kienböck disease to be 0.27%, with 0.10% being incidental findings and 0.17% in symptomatic individuals.[19] In the study, younger patients (mean age 43 years) with more advanced carpal collapse were more likely to be symptomatic than older patients (mean age 54 years) who were in precollapse stages of disease.[19] In Kienböck original series, most patients were male laborers between the age of 20 and 29 years.[5] Since that time, larger studies have supported a male predominance with a male to female ratio of 2 to 4:1[2].

Recent studies have also suggested a possible genetic component to Kienböck disease. Kazmers and colleagues identified familial enrichment and an increased relative risk of Kienböck disease among first-degree relatives, although the specific genetic mutations remain unknown.[20] Risk factors in that study that correlated with the development of Kienböck disease included diabetes, alcohol and tobacco use, and prolonged corticosteroid use.[20]

Since Kienböck original description of "lunatomalacia" in 1910, manual laborers have been found to have the highest incidence of Kienböck disease. In fact, in 1920 Walter Mueller coined the term "occupational lunatomalacia" to describe the pathologic changes to the lunate in Kienböck disease from repetitive overload.[21] This was later supported in larger series by Stahl (1947) and Therkelson (1949) where over 97% of patients with Kienböck disease were found to be manual laborers.[22,23]

In addition to manual laborers, individuals with cerebral palsy (CP) have also previously been shown to have a relatively high incidence of Kienböck disease. This is believed to be associated with spasticity, habitual wrist flexion, and subsequent volar vascular injury.[24] In a series of adult CP patients living in an assisted living facility, Rooker and colleagues found 5 of 53 residents (9%) to have radiographic evidence of Kienböck disease.[24] Other reports have shown the incidence of Kienböck disease in patients with CP to be between 2% and 10%, with unique disease manifestations associated with spastic CP such as bilateral involvement as well as unilateral Kienböck disease affecting the nondominant hand.[25,26]

Another population thought to have a higher predilection for developing Kienböck disease is athletes. Nakamura and colleagues investigated the difference in age and sex distribution, symptoms, and radiographic findings between 91 cases of Kienböck disease related to sports and manual labor.[27] The authors found that athletes participating in tennis, handball, and Asian martial arts had similar clinical and radiographic findings as manual laborers but had a significantly shorter period of insult before the onset of symptoms (5 vs 9 years on average).[27]

CLINICAL PRESENTATION

The typical Kienböck disease patient is a manual laborer with unilateral activity-related complaints affecting the dominant wrist.[8] History of known previous traumatic event is variable.

Nonspecific symptoms are often reported, including generalized central wrist pain, dorsal wrist swelling, and pain with grip, loading, and decreased range of motion.[2] Grip strength may be decreased up to 50% of the contralateral side.[28] Dorsal wrist pain is often worse with wrist extension. Percussion of the third metacarpal head with the patient's handheld in a fist has been described to elicit pain over the lunate.[1]

The radiographic workup for suspected Kienböck disease involves 3 views of the wrist (AP, lateral, and 45° oblique). Ulnar variance views are also important to assess for possible ulnar impaction syndrome in the ulnar positive wrist. Although ulnar negative variance has historically been associated with Kienböck disease, its exact role in the etiology of Kienböck disease is now considered more controversial.[29] Nonetheless, radial shortening in the setting of ulnar negative patients with early Kienböck disease remains popular as studies have shown consistently reduced radiolunate contact pressure and improved healing with this symptomatology.[30,31]

Radiographs are typically normal in early disease but help to differentiate between other sources of dorsal wrist pain, including fracture, ulnolunate impaction, carpal instability, and arthritis. Sclerosis of the lunate is an early finding that correlates with osteonecrosis. In the later stages of Kienböck disease, plain radiographs will reveal progression of lunate collapse, fracture, scaphoid flexion, loss of carpal height, and carpal arthritis.[2]

Advanced imaging is often required for accurate staging and surgical planning. CT scans provide better detail of the osseous architecture than plain films and are able to detect subtle lunate fractures and collapse. Micro-CT has previously been used experimentally to detect unique microstructural differences in lunate morphology compared with normal bone. Recently, Han and colleagues found lunate changes in patients with advanced Kienböck disease to result in thicker, denser, and flatter trabeculae in response to internal stress.[32] This plate-like microstructure identified on CT corresponded to areas of osteonecrosis identified on radiographs and MRI, sclerotic and dead bone on histology, and is hypothesized to limit reparative mesenchymal stem cell migration.[32]

MRI scans are helpful early in the disease process where plain radiographs appear normal. Early findings of Kienböck disease on MRI include diffuse hyperintensity of the lunate on T1 imaging. Later findings include diffuse hypointensity of the lunate on T1 and T2 sequences, indicating decreased vascularity. This helps to distinguish Kienböck disease from ulnolunate impaction syndrome, which is typically hyperintense on T2 sequences secondary to bone edema at the point of impaction in proximal lunate and nonprogressive. Gadolinium-enhanced MRI scans are a helpful adjunct to T1 fat-suppressed imaging and have been shown to improve diagnostic accuracy and assist in surgical planning.[2,33] Schmitt and colleagues have previously described areas of increased gadolinium enhancement are thought to represent neovascular tissue with increased reparative potential whereas areas of decreased enhancement are thought to represent bone edema (**Table 2**).[33,34]

In addition to CT and MRI, wrist arthroscopy is an additional diagnostic tool to assess the integrity of the chondral surface of the lunate as well as its adjacent carpal articulations.[35] During arthroscopy, the lunate and perilunate surfaces are inspected for chondral damage or fracture, as well as softening, chondral flaps/defects, concealed lesions, and degeneration.[36] Loose osteochondral fragments, flaps, and synovitis are debrided and "functional articulations" can be identified for later reconstruction.[36] Proponents of wrist arthroscopy have found that articular damage is underestimated on plain imaging, findings on arthroscopy usually lead to a change in management plan, and some cases have an intact chondral surface despite subchondral compromise on advanced imaging.[35,36] This led to the development of the arthroscopy-based Bain and Begg classification system of Kienböck disease, which helps surgeons determine the appropriate surgical treatment plan where "nonfunctional articular surfaces" can bypassed or excised to reduce pain and maintain functional wrist movement (**Table 3**).[35]

TREATMENT TRENDS

Historically, the treatment of Kienböck disease was largely conservative. In Kienböck 1910 manuscript, he advocated for splint immobilization for symptom control in most patients and lunate excision reserved for patients only in advanced stages with recalcitrant pain.[1] Although early lunate excision did have some early proponents,[1] conservative treatment remained the predominant treatment philosophy until the association of negative ulnar variance with Kienböck disease was elucidated in 1928 by Hulten.[7] This led to the emergence of joint leveling procedures such as radial shortening and ulnar lengthening[37] in the 1940s. Later, intercarpal fusions in the 1960s,[38] capitate shortening in the 1980s,[39,40] and radial wedge osteotomy in the 1990s[41] followed to decrease stress across the lunate and permit healing.

Table 2
Schmitt classification of lunate vascularity

Pattern	MRI Findings	Prognosis
A	Homogenous enhancement of lunate with bone marrow edema; intact lunate perfusion	Good
B	Heterogenous signal with enhancement of the reparative zone and visible distal bone; partial osteonecrosis	Intermediate
C	No contrast enhancement; complete osteonecrosis	Poor

Adapted from Lichtman DM, Pientka WF, Bain GI. Kienböck Disease: Moving Forward. J Hand Surg. 2016;41(5):630-638. https://doi.org/10.1016/j.jhsa.2016.02.013; with permission.

Table 3
Bain and Begg arthroscopic classification of Kienböck disease

Grade	Nonfunctional Articulation
0	None
1	Lp
2A	Lp/R
2B	Lp/Ld
3	R/Lp/Ld C is typically spared
4	R/Lp/Ld/C

Abbreviations: C, proximal capitate articular surface; Ld, distal lunate; Lp, proximal lunate; R, lunate facet of radius.

Adapted from Bain GI, Begg M. Arthroscopic assessment and classification of Kienbock's disease. *Tech Hand Up Extrem Surg.* 2006;10(1):8-13. https://doi.org/10.1097/00130911-200603000-00003; with permission.

However, until the 1970s, the treatment of advanced Kienböck disease remained problematic, as lunate excision was the only surgical option. This often resulted in significant carpal shift and shortening. In 1970, Swanson attempted to solve this problem by filling the void after lunate excision with a silicone interposition arthroplasty. In his patients, this achieved good long-term functional results.[42,43] However, because of issues with silicone-associated synovitis, this technique was later abandoned. That same year, Nahigian developed a dorsal flap interposition arthroplasty, which resulted in symptomatic improvement for all 4 patients in his series, and prevention of carpal migration.[44]

In the 1990s and 2000s, significant interest emerged in developing techniques to restore lunate vascularity in early and more advanced disease. For early disease, both distal radius and ulna core decompression,[45] as well as direct lunate core decompression,[46] were described to relieve increased intraosseous pressure and incite a local inflammatory/healing response. In addition, multiple techniques of pedicled corticoperiosteal vascularized bone flaps from adjacent bones were developed for patients without secondary arthritis.[47] This idea was based on previous work by Hori who demonstrated in a canine study that transplantation of a vascular bundle into necrotic bone resulted in neovascularization and bone growth.[48] Although these procedures relieve pain in most patients and demonstrate modest improvements in wrist range of motion, they are unable to reverse radiographic changes or replace degenerate cartilage.[49] This limitation of pedicled vascularized bone grafts ultimately inspired the application of free vascularized osteochondral flaps from the medial femoral trochlea for restoration of lunate height, vascularity, and chondral deficiency in advanced Kienböck disease.[49]

Currently, there are over 20 procedures described for the treatment of Kienböck disease.[16] In a recent survey of 375 American Society for Surgery of the Hand (ASSH) members, Danoff and colleagues found that for early disease, the most popular treatments for Kienböck were splint/cast immobilization or radial shortening osteotomy.[50] Kolovich and colleagues in a similar survey study found a high acceptance (29%) of distal radius core decompression for stage I disease.[51] In the setting of lunate collapse without fixed scaphoid rotation (stage IIIa), radial shortening osteotomy was most performed in the setting of negative ulnar variance, whereas vascularized bone flap or capitate shortening osteotomy was performed in the setting of ulnar positive variance. For vascular bone grafting, a technique utilizing the fourth and fifth extensor compartment was most popular in a separate survey of fellowship-trained hand surgeons.[51] In the setting of lunate collapse with fixed scaphoid rotation (stage IIIb), salvage procedures such as proximal row carpectomy or limited intercarpal arthrodesis were most commonly used. Lastly, when carpal collapse was present, as well as significant adjacent carpal arthritis (stage IV), proximal row carpectomy or total wrist fusion was most common.[50] The lack of consensus surrounding Kienböck disease treatment is a testament to the need for new long-term comparative studies to determine optimal management for the disease for all stages.

SUMMARY

Over a century has passed since Kienböck description of lunate osteonecrosis. In that time, improvements in imaging technology such as CT and MRI have enabled a better understanding of changes in the osseous architecture and vascularity of the lunate over time in patients with the disease. In addition, the advent of wrist arthroscopy has enabled more accurate assessment of the lunate chondral surface, and thereby facilitated more precise treatment planning. However, despite these great strides in our understanding, there is still significant uncertainty regarding the pathogenesis of Kienböck disease and the optimal methods for treatment because of the rarity of the disease and lack of prospective long-term comparative studies.[2]

- Kienböck disease is a rare disease primarily affecting the dominant wrist of male laborers aged 20 to 40 years
- Presentation is variable and often delayed
- Etiology of Kienböck disease includes mechanical and biological factors
- Improvements in advanced imaging technology and wrist arthroscopy have allowed for more accurate staging and strategic surgical planning
- Treatment today is based on integrity of chondral surfaces, lunate structural integrity, and vascular supply, as well as age of the patient

CLINICS CARE POINTS

- Kienböck disease is a rare but clinically important source of activity-related dorsal wrist pain in younger adults
- Early diagnosis allows for less invasive surgical techniques that maintain wrist motion

- Advanced imaging and wrist arthroscopy are helpful to assess the osseous, vascular, and chondral anatomy to optimize surgical approach and outcome

DISCLOSURE

The authors have nothing to disclose.

REFERENCES

1. Gerwin M. The history of Kienböck's disease. Hand Clin 1993;9(3):385–90.
2. Rioux-Forker D, Shin AY. Osteonecrosis of the Lunate: Kienböck Disease. J Am Acad Orthop Surg 2020;28(14):570–84.
3. Wagner JP, Chung KC. A historical report on Robert Kienböck (1871-1953) and Kienböck's Disease. J Hand Surg 2005;30(6):1117–21.
4. Chochole M. Robert Kienbock: the man and his work. J Hand Surg Eur 2010;35(7):534–7.
5. Kilnböck R. The Classic: Concerning Traumatic Malacia of the Lunate and its Consequences: Degeneration and Compression Fractures. Clin Orthop Relat Res 1980;149:4–8.
6. Goldsmith R. KIENBÖCH'S DISEASE OF THE SEMI-LUNAR BONE. Ann Surg 1925;81(4):857–62.
7. Hulten O. Uber Anatomische Variationen der Handgelenkknochen. Acta Radiol 1928;9(2):155–68.
8. Schuind F, Eslami S, Ledoux P. Kienböck's disease. J Bone Joint Surg Br 2008;90-B(2):133–9.
9. Durbin FC. The early changes of Kienböck's disease of the carpal lunate bone. Proc R Soc Med 1951;44(6):482–8.
10. Lichtman DM, Pientka WF, Bain GI. Kienböck Disease: A New Algorithm for the 21st Century. J Wrist Surg 2017;6(1):2–10.
11. Kennedy C, Abrams R. In Brief: The Lichtman Classification for Kienböck Disease. Clin Orthop 2019;477(6):1516–20.
12. Jafarnia K, Collins ED, Kohl HW, et al. Reliability of the Lichtman classification of Kienböck's disease. J Hand Surg 2000;25(3):529–34.
13. Gelberman RH, Bauman TD, Menon J, et al. The vascularity of the lunate bone and Kienböck's disease. J Hand Surg 1980;5(3):272–8.
14. Dubey PP, Chauhan NK, Siddiqui MS, et al. Study of vascular supply of lunate and consideration applied to Kienböck disease. Hand Surg 2011;16(1):9–13.
15. Jensen CH. Intraosseous pressure in Kienböck's disease. J Hand Surg 1993;18(2):355–9.
16. Squitieri L, Petruska E, Chung KC. Publication bias in Kienböck's disease: systematic review. J Hand Surg 2010;35(3):359–67.e5.
17. Mennen U, Sithebe H. The incidence of asymptomatic Kienböck's disease. J Hand Surg Eur 2009;34(3):348–50.
18. Tsujimoto R, Maeda J, Abe Y, et al. Epidemiology of Kienböck's disease in middle-aged and elderly Japanese women. Orthopedics 2015;38(1):e14–8.
19. van Leeuwen WF, Janssen SJ, ter Meulen DP, et al. What Is the Radiographic Prevalence of Incidental Kienböck Disease? Clin Orthop 2016;474(3):808–13.
20. Kazmers NH, Yu Z, Barker T, et al. Evaluation for Kienböck Disease Familial Clustering: A Population-Based Cohort Study. J Hand Surg 2020;45(1):1–8.e1.
21. Irisarri C. Aetiology of Kienböck's Disease. Handchir Mikrochir Plast Chir 2010;42(03):157–61.
22. Ståhl F, Brown LJ. On Lunatomalacia (Kienböck's Disease): A Clinical and Roentgenological Study, Especially on Its Pathogenesis and Late Results of Immobilization Treatment. Acta Chir Scand, (Supplementum)1947;126:1–133.
23. Therkelsen F, Andersen K. Lunatomalacia. Acta Chir Scand 1949;97(6):503–26.
24. Rooker GD, Goodfellow JW. Kienböck's disease in cerebral palsy. J Bone Joint Surg Br 1977;59(3):363–5.
25. Joji S, Mizuseki T, Katayama S, et al. Aetiology of Kienböck's disease based on a study of the condition among patients with cerebral palsy. J Hand Surg Edinb Scotl 1993;18(3):294–8.
26. Gallien P, Candelier G, Nicolas B, et al. Kienböck's disease and cerebral palsy case report. Ann Phys Rehabil Med 2010;53(2):118–23.
27. Nakamura R, Imaeda T, Suzuki K, et al. Sports-related Kienböck's disease. Am J Sports Med 1991;19(1):88–91.
28. Cross D, Matullo KS. Kienböck Disease. Orthop Clin North Am 2014;45(1):141–52.
29. D'Hoore K, De Smet L, Verellen K, et al. Negative ulnar variance is not a risk factor for Kienböck's disease. J Hand Surg 1994;19(2):229–31.
30. Žiger T, Kopljar M, Bakota B, et al. Experimental shortening of the radius in the treatment of Kienböck's disease. Injury 2020;S0020-1383(20):30110–8.
31. Weiss AP. Radial shortening. Hand Clin 1993;9(3):475–82.
32. Han KJ, Kim JY, Chung NS, et al. Trabecular microstructure of the human lunate in Kienböck's disease. J Hand Surg Eur 2012;37(4):336–41.
33. Lichtman DM, Pientka WF, Bain GI. Kienböck Disease: Moving Forward. J Hand Surg 2016;41(5):630–8.
34. Schmitt R, Heinze A, Fellner F, et al. Imaging and staging of avascular osteonecroses at the wrist and hand. Eur J Radiol 1997;25(2):92–103.
35. Bain GI, Begg M. Arthroscopic assessment and classification of Kienböck's disease. Tech Hand Up Extrem Surg 2006;10(1):8–13.

36. MacLean SBM, Kantar K, Bain GI, et al. The Role of Wrist Arthroscopy in Kienbock Disease. Hand Clin 2017;33(4):727–34.

37. Persson M. Causal treatment of lunatomalacia; further experiences of operative ulna lengthening. Acta Chir Scand 1950;100(6):531–44.

38. Graner O, Lopes EI, Carvalho BC, et al. Arthrodesis of the Carpal Bones in the Treatment of Kienböck's Disease, Painful Ununited Fractures of the Navicular and Lunate Bones with Avascular Necrosis, and Old Fracture-Dislocations of Carpal Bones. JBJS 1966; 48(4):767–74.

39. Almquist EE. Kienbock's disease. Clin Orthop 1986;(202):68–78.

40. Almquist EE. Capitate shortening in the treatment of Kienböck's disease. Hand Clin 1993;9(3):505–12.

41. Nakamura R, Tsuge S, Watanabe K, et al. Radial wedge osteotomy for Kienböck disease. JBJS 1991;73(9):1391–6.

42. Swanson AB. Silicone rubber implants for the replacement of the carpal scaphoid and lunate bones. Orthop Clin North Am 1970;1(2):299–309.

43. Swanson AB, Maupin BK, de Groot Swanson G, et al. Lunate implant resection arthroplasty: Long-term results. J Hand Surg 1985;10(6, Part 2):1013–24.

44. Nahigian SH, Li CS, Richey DG, et al. The Dorsal Flap Arthroplasty in the Treatment of Kienböck's Disease. JBJS 1970;52(2):245–52.

45. Illarramendi AA, Schulz C, De Carli P. The surgical treatment of Kienböck's disease by radius and ulna metaphyseal core decompression. J Hand Surg 2001;26(2):252–60.

46. Mehrpour SR, Kamrani RS, Aghamirsalim MR, et al. Treatment of Kienböck disease by lunate core decompression. J Hand Surg 2011;36(10):1675–7.

47. Shin AY, Bishop AT, Berger RA. Vascularized Pedicled Bone Grafts for Disorders of the Carpus. Tech Hand Up Extrem Surg 1998;2(2):94–109.

48. Hori Y, Tamai S, Okuda H, et al. Blood vessel transplantation to bone. J Hand Surg 1979;4(1):23–33.

49. Bürger HK, Windhofer C, Gaggl AJ, et al. Vascularized medial femoral trochlea osteochondral flap reconstruction of advanced Kienböck disease. J Hand Surg 2014;39(7):1313–22.

50. Danoff JR, Cuellar DO, Jane O, et al. The Management of Kienböck Disease: A Survey of the ASSH Membership. J Wrist Surg 2015;4(1):43–8.

51. Kolovich GP, Kalu CMK, Ruff ME. Current Trends in Treatment of Kienböck Disease. Hand N Y N 2016; 11(1):113–8.

The Pathoanatomy and Biomechanics of Kienböck Disease

Simon B.M. MacLean, MBChB, FRCS(Tr&Orth), PGDipCE[a],*,
Minhao Hu, BClinSc, MD, MSurg[b],
Gregory I. Bain, PhD, MBBS, FRACS, , FA(Ortho)A[c]

KEYWORDS

● Kienböck disease ● Etiology ● Pathogenesis ● Dynamic ● Instability

KEY POINTS

● The etiology and pathogenesis of Kienböck disease involves osseous, vascular, and chondral aspects of the lunate and the wrist, including the proximal and distal articulations with the radius and capitate, respectively.
● There is not one typical "Kienböck's phenotype"; disease can be seen both in the young and the elderly, in both sexes, and radiographic progression may differ in each group
● Dynamic" pathology is seen at different stages of Kienböck disease. Dynamic pathology can contribute to symptoms and is important for disease progression. We recommend 4-dimensional computed tomography scanning in select cases to determine these dynamic aspects of the disease.

INTRODUCTION

Since its original description in 1910, Kienböck disease (KD) has remained an enigma.[1] The disease is rare, and many widely held views on etiology and the "at-risk" patient stem from historical observational studies.[2,3] Much of this landmark work has become dogma among hand surgeons, but many of these key findings have failed to be reproduced in later studies.[4,5] There is a lack of clarity, therefore, as to the precise etiology and pathogenesis of the disease. As a consequence, the optimum management of the disease remains a source of debate.

The lunate is regarded as the "keystone" of the wrist and is essential for the stable equilibrium required for normal wrist kinematics. Integrity of the lunate requires biological and mechanical homeostasis, allowing load transfer and function as the intercalated segment in the proximal row of the carpus. When this "keystone" is compromised, lunate fracture, collapse, and degeneration of the wrist can occur. The progression of the disease, however, is variable and the natural history debated.[6,7]

We present our theories on the etiology and pathogenesis of KD, based on basic science models, previous literature, personal case experience, and static and *dynamic* imaging, using our kinematic observations of the Kienböck wrist.[7–9]

THE "AT-RISK" WRIST FOR KIENBÖCK DISEASE
The Patient

The "at-risk" Kienböck's demographic was traditionally thought to be a male, manual laborer, between 20 and 40 years of age, with the dominant limb affected. This is an overly simplified view, however, as there is no "typical" Kienböck's

a Department of Orthopaedic Surgery, Tauranga Hospital, 829 Cameron Road South, Bay of Plenty, Tauranga, North Island 3112, New Zealand; b Department of Plastic and Reconstructive Surgery, Flinders Medical Centre, Adelaide, South Australia 5042, Australia; c Hand and Upper Limb Surgery, Flinders University, Bedford Park, Adelaide, South Australia 5042, Australia
* Corresponding author.
E-mail address: Simonmaclean81@gmail.com

Hand Clin 38 (2022) 393–403
https://doi.org/10.1016/j.hcl.2022.03.003
0749-0712/22/© 2022 Elsevier Inc. All rights reserved.

patient. The disease can present at any age, in either sex, and can be associated with other conditions.

THE 3 PHENOTYPES OF KIENBÖCK DISEASE

We have recently performed a systematic review on the natural radiographic progression of Kienböck disease following nonoperative treatment. We have made a number of observations that challenge previous dogma on the disease, including the following:

- A greater proportion of women aged older than 60 years were diagnosed compared with men (n = 28, 39% vs n = 7, 9%).
- In patients older than 34 years at diagnosis, a positive ulnar variance (n = 25) was more common than ulnar-neutral (n = 15) or ulnar-negative variance (n = 10).
- There was no significant difference in progression observed between patients when comparing dominant versus nondominant hands.

From these observations, and those of other investigators, we propose that there are 3 phenotypes of KD:

1. The young "*Teenbock*" patient, with disease that is usually self-limiting.
2. The typical "*middle-aged male manual worker*," with negative ulnar variance.
3. The "*older female*" patient, often with positive ulnar variance. These patients may have ulnocarpal impaction *and* KD, or have only ulnocarpal impaction *in isolation* having been misdiagnosed with KD.

The rate of radiographic progression in older patients (59 years and older) is higher (*P* < .001) (**Fig. 1**). Female patients also tend to have a higher rate of radiographic progression compared with male patients (*P* < .001) (**Fig. 2**).

MEDICAL CONDITIONS

KD has also been reported with arterial diseases such as endarteritis, thrombotic disorders such as sickle cell anemia, diver's decompression disease from nitrogen bubbles within the lunate, cerebral palsy, and steroid medications. The disease also has been reported within families.[10–15]

THE LUNATE
Lunate: Osseous Factors

The lunate is regarded as the "keystone" of the wrist, and transfers load via the central column of

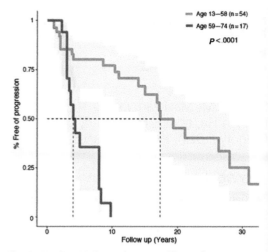

Fig. 1. Kaplan-Meier estimates; effect of age on progression of KD. (*Courtesy of* Greg Bain, PhD, MBBS, FRACS, FA(Ortho)A, Adelaide, Australia).

the wrist from the capitate to the lunate and through the lunate to the distal radius. It is the intercalated segment of the proximal row, with only the volar and dorsal capsules and interosseous ligaments inserting onto it.

Viegas-Type Lunates

Lunate morphology plays a role. Viegas-type 1 lunates are more common in KD. They are small, trapezoidal and have intraosseous trabecular angulation exceeding 135°. They tend to preferentially load through the mid-carpal joint in contrast to type 2 lunates, which load through the radiocarpal joint.[8,16] Type 1 lunates do not have an articular

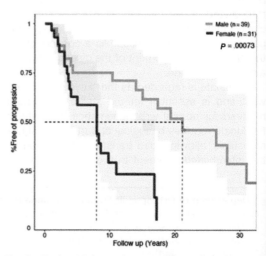

Fig. 2. Kaplan-Meier estimates; effect of sex on progression of KD. (*Courtesy of* Greg Bain, PhD, MBBS, FRACS, FA(Ortho)A, Adelaide, Australia).

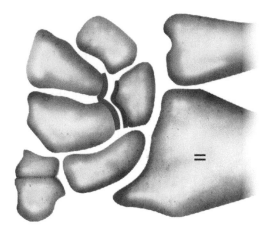

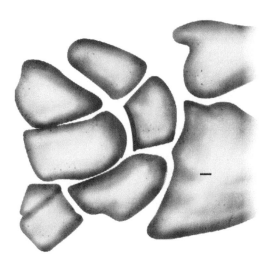

Fig. 3. Viegas type 1 and type 2 lunates.

facet for the hamate and therefore point-load between the capitate and distal radius, which may increase susceptibility for stress fracture (**Fig. 3**).

Zapico-Type Lunates

Zapico's[17] observations were similar. He classified lunates into 3 groups based on osseous differences. He found that his trapezoidal "type 1" lunates were more susceptible to KD and hypothesized that this was due to trabecular geometry creating a "plane of weakness," together with a higher prevalence of ulnar-negative variance.[17] The "wedge" shape of the Zapico type-1 lunate is also likely to contribute. Load from the capitate is likely to be transferred as shear rather than axial forces through the subchondral bone plate. With trabeculae being less resistant to shear forces, this may increase susceptibility to fracture through the lunate.

Micro-computed tomography (CT) demonstrates that the proximal subchondral bone plate of the lunate is only a single layer thick, making it more vulnerable to stress fracture.[18,19] This is consistent with our observation of fracture mapping in KD lunates, that most of the subchondral bone plate fractures occur proximally rather than distally (**Fig. 4**).

Ulnar-negative variance increases load on the radial half of the lunate, as the ulnar half of the bone tends to overhang the edge of the radius. Historical studies observed a significant association between KD and negative ulnar variance, although this finding has failed to be reproduced in later studies.[2,4,5]

Our dynamic CT study supports some of these findings.[8] Most patients in our study had Viegas type-1 lunates (23 of 24) and had ulnar-negative variance (18 of 24).[8] We hypothesize that negative ulnar variance, particularly in combination with a

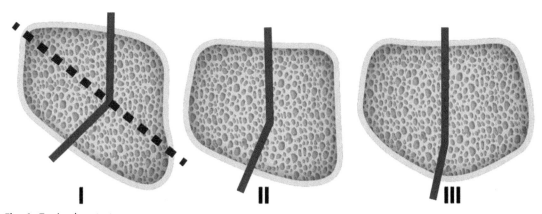

Fig. 4. Zapico lunate types.

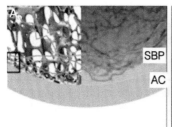
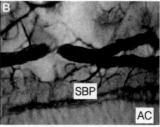

Fig. 5. Subarticular venous plexus of the lunate. (*A*) A composite image of subarticular venous plexus and 3D micro-CT of the subchondral bone plate. The small box on the left of the image depicts the area demonstrated in the magnified views shown in (*B*), where the venule within the subarticular plexus is seen in profile. The calcified zone of the AC, and SBP are well seen. 3D, 3-dimensional; AC, articular cartilage; CT, computed tomography; SBP, subchondral bone plate. (*Courtesy of* H. Crock, AO, Victoria, Australia).

type-1 lunate, further increases axial load and shear forces through the lunate, increasing susceptibility for stress fracture. We believe a critical factor is that the lunate is uncovered over the ulnar edge of the distal radius, and the proximal and distal surfaces are exposed to a cantilever effect between the capitate and the radius. Fatigue failure of the lunate occurs as an impaction fracture, on the single-layered proximal subchondral bone plate, at the point where the most ulnar aspect of the distal radius impinges on the proximal lunate.

Lunate: Vascular Factors

Arterial flow to the lunate is limited to only the volar and dorsal aspects. There is a network of 5 named arteries, which include the radial, ulnar, anterior, deep palmar, and dorsal arteries. These arteries form a network and divide into 3 volar and 3 dorsal transverse arches. Supply through the volar aspect is predominant, and is less consistent dorsally. Intraosseous vascularity patterns were reported by Lee,[20] and later Gelberman and

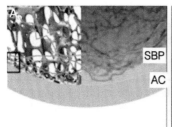

Copyright Dr Gregory Bain

Fig. 6. Compartment syndrome of bone. Diagrammatic representation of the normal vascularization of the lunate (superior half) with the normal fat cells and venous drainage. With ischemia (inferior half), there is interstitial edema and the marrow fat cells become swollen. This leads to tamponade of the sinusoids, thus decreasing the venous outflow. This further increases the intraosseous pressure, reducing arterial inflow and produces necrosis. (*Courtesy of* Greg Bain, PhD, MBBS, FRACS, FA(Ortho)A, Adelaide, Australia).

Bauman.[21] They hypothesized that a single volar artery may predispose to KD.[20,21] It is worth noting, however, that avascular necrosis of the lunate secondary to trauma, such as translunate fracture dislocation, is rare.

Venous factors may be more important in the etiology of KD. Crock[22] studied the venous drainage of the lunate, describing the extraosseous veins that accompany the arteries and the subarticular venous plexus, below the subchondral bone plate (**Fig. 5**).

Literature supports impairment of venous drainage as critical in the development of avascular necrosis in the lunate and femoral head.[23] We also know that increased intraosseous pressure in the lunate is seen in KD and rises significantly on wrist extension.[24] Jensen[25] hypothesized that impairment in venous outflow may be factor in the development of KD.

Two mechanisms may lead to venous obstruction: producing either a *localized* or *global* phenomenon. Obstruction of a single vein will produce a global hypertension of the lunate. A stress fracture of the proximal lunate will violate the subarticular venous plexus and produce localized venous hypertension, producing edema of the fat cells, increasing the intraosseous hypertension. This further reduces arterial inflow, leading to an *intraosseous compartment syndrome* and osseous necrosis (**Fig. 6**).[7]

There is an interesting group of patients who present with sclerosis of the entire lunate. This corresponds to the Lichtman type 1, and the Schmitt B.[26] We postulate that the entire lunate is compromised, due to obstruction of the volar venous drainage (**Fig. 7**).

THE "AT-RISK" WRIST FOR COLLAPSE

Although osseous and vascular factors remain important, we know that not every KD wrist develops carpal collapse. There is a paucity of literature on the natural history of the condition, which remains unclear. Our work reviewing the dynamic

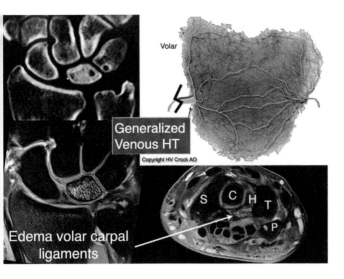

Fig. 7. Edema of the volar carpal ligaments (*arrow*), leading to generalized venous hypertension (HT) obstruction of the venous drainage of the entire lunate. S, scaphoid; C, capitate; H, hamate; T, triquetrum; P, pisiform. (*Courtesy of* H. Crock, AO, Victoria, Australia).

motion of patients with Kienböck's using 4-dimensional (4D) CT scanning has highlighted mechanical dynamic aspects of the disease that may be important for disease progression. There are a number of pathologies diagnosed only on dynamic imaging. We term these "dynamic pathologies," and when present, can become symptomatic in isolation or contribute to fracture and collapse of the lunate. These are outlined as follows.

Fractures of the Lunate

Study of fracture morphology within the lunate aids in understanding the pathogenesis of collapse and instability in the Kienböck wrist. The coronal lunate fracture in KD has already been well-described. Of equal prevalence, we have identified a *sagittal* fracture line through the lunate seen on dynamic 4D-CT coronal images. We

believe this fracture to result from the "nutcracker phenomenon," corresponding to point loading through the ulnar edge of the radius, leading to a lunate impaction fracture.[7]

In our study, *lunate ligament attachment fractures* were seen in nearly half of our cases, in both early and late disease. They represent detachment or avulsion of the interosseous ligaments or extrinsic carpal ligaments attached to the lunate.

Subchondral bone plate fractures occur both proximally and distally. Arthroscopically, these may be identified on probing of the lunate in the presence of an intact articular surface. In these cases, on ballottement, a "floating" articular surface is identified.[27–29]

We have recently mapped fracture lines on CT scan in patients with KD (**Fig. 8**). The coronal fracture is often considered to occur in isolation. We

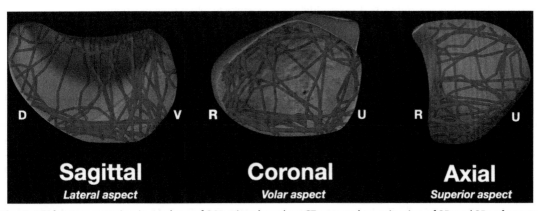

Fig. 8. KD fracture mapping in a cohort of 24 patient based on CT scan and examination of 2D and 3D reformats. D, dorsal; V, volar; R, radial; U, ulnar. (*Courtesy of* Simon MacLean, MBChB, FRCS(Tr&Orth), PGDipCE, North Island, New Zealand).

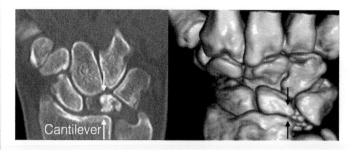

Fig. 9. Coronal 2D CT image and 3D CT image from the dorsal aspect. White and black arrows represent the loading point of the lunate between the capitate and radius. (*Courtesy of* Greg Bain, PhD, MBBS, FRACS, FA(Ortho)A, Adelaide, Australia and Simon MacLean, MBChB, FRCS(Tr&Orth), PGDipCE, North Island, New Zealand).

have found that coronal and sagittal fracture lines *rarely* occur in isolation and are usually associated with fractures to the subchondral bone plates, proximally or distally, and avulsion of the ligament attachments.

- *Sagittal view*: Coronal fractures are distributed throughout the lunate, but most coronal fractures occur in the *volar horn* of the lunate. Most subchondral bone plate fractures occur proximally.
- *Coronal view*: Ligament attachment fractures at the lunotriquetral and scapholunate insertions are common. The proximal subchondral bone plate fractures are commonly seen.
- *Axial view*: Most coronal fractures are throughout the *volar horn*.

Dynamic Factors

The nutcracker effect

We define the "nutcracker effect" as *dynamic proximal capitate migration through a fractured lunate causing fragment separation*. This can be seen on dynamic sagittal 2D images with wrist flexion and extension and 2D coronal images with the wrist in radial and ulnar deviation (**Fig. 9**). The nutcracker effect is a consequence of the capitate loading on a Viegas type-1 lunate with ulnar-negative variance. The proximal capitate point-loads on a small trapezoidal lunate with an oblique distal articular surface. Central column axial forces through the capitate are transferred as shear forces and point loading occurs on the ulnar edge of the distal radius, which acts as a fulcrum. Cantilever loading of the lunate is exacerbated by ulnar and radial deviation of the wrist, and the lunate becomes "hinged" over the ulnar edge of the radius. This hinging leads to repetitive point loading, and the lunate fails to translate across the distal radial articular surface with motion. This "nutcracker" effect was present in 15 (75%) of 20 patients in our study, and found to be highly associated with a sagittal fracture

line corresponding to the point of loading among the radius, lunate, and capitate.[8]

VOLAR RADIOLUNATE IMPINGEMENT

In our long-term outcome study, we found that coronal fracture of the lunate was a poor prognostic indicator for a lunate salvage procedure, as it usually precedes lunate collapse and fragmentation.[9] On dynamic sagittal images, with coronal lunate fractures, we have identified that the volar horn of the lunate remains static in wrist extension, with its volar radiolunate ligament attachments. With wrist flexion, the capitate translates anteriorly and tilts the volar horn of the lunate, creating mechanical impingement over the volar rim of the distal radius. We term this "volar radiolunate impingement," and have found it to be associated with advanced stages of the disease (**Fig. 10**). This finding is important to identify, as it may be a cause of persistent symptoms following surgery. We have found it to be associated with advanced stages of the disease.[8] Separation of the volar horn fragment with the corresponding ligament attachments of the short and long radiolunate ligaments, and scapholunate and lunotriquetral ligaments can lead to proximal row instability (dynamic or static), and radiocarpal instability (ulnar translocation).

ULNAR STYLOID TRIQUETRAL IMPINGEMENT

Ulnar styloid impaction syndrome is usually associated with a morphologically long ulnar styloid or an ulnar styloid nonunion.[30] We have found it to be a common finding in advanced stages of KD, associated with decreasing carpal height, ulnar translocation, and carpal collapse. These patients often have ulnar-sided wrist pain, particularly with ulnar deviation. Correcting carpal height with reconstructive motion-preserving surgery can disimpact the triquetrum, leading to improvement in ulnar-sided symptoms (**Fig. 11**). Ulnar styloid triquetral impingement may be a cause of ulnar-sided wrist pain in patients with advanced stages of KD.[8]

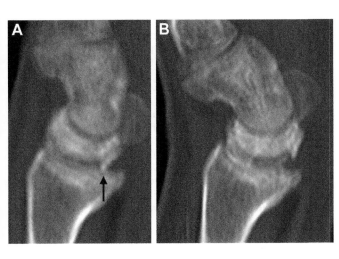

Fig. 10. Volar radiolunate impingement. Sagittal CT scan images. Note how the volar horn remains separate from the lunate fossa in extension (*A*) but impinges on the volar lunate facet in wrist flexion (*B*). (*Courtesy of* Greg Bain, PhD, MBBS, FRACS, FA(Ortho)A, Adelaide, Australia and Simon MacLean, MBChB, FRCS(Tr&Orth), PGDipCE, North Island, New Zealand).

INSTABILITY PATTERNS IN KIENBÖCK DISEASE

Instability of the carpus in KD is a complex phenomenon. The intrinsic (interosseous) and extrinsic (radiocarpal) ligaments can be affected through attenuation, rupture, or avulsion. Compromise of these restraints in isolation or combination can lead to different patterns of instability. Instability can occur (1) within the lunate (internal), (2) within the proximal row (intrinsic), or (3) between the radius and the carpus (extrinsic). Instability can be static (diagnosed on static imaging) or dynamic (diagnosed on wrist motion on dynamic CT scanning). We expand on these concepts and their etiology in the following section.

Dynamic Proximal Row Instability

We have shown that interosseous ligament tears in the proximal row are frequently found at arthroscopy in patients with KD.[9] Scapholunate and lunotriquetral instability can occur by 2 mechanisms: (1) attenuation and rupture, or (2) fracture of the lunate adjacent to the ligament attachments. Dynamic instability of the proximal row is defined as

scapholunate or lunotriquetral instability diagnosed through wrist motion on dynamic 4D-CT scanning. Dynamic instability may precede static instability on static imaging, and precedes carpal collapse. Strategies used to salvage or bypass the lunate should take into consideration the status of the interosseous ligaments. As well as the classic coronal fracture, ligament avulsion fractures should be identified on CT scan, as these may represent instability of the proximal carpal row.[8]

Internal Instability of the Lunate

Dynamic assessment of KD kinematics shows separation of lunate fracture fragments depending on the forces applied and wrist position. On examination of dynamic sagittal imaging, the volar and dorsal horns move independently of each other with wrist flexion and extension. On dynamic coronal sequences, the radial and ulnar lunate fragments move independently with radial and ulnar deviation and clenched-fist loading. We have termed this phenomenon "internal instability of the lunate" (**Fig. 12**). This finding illustrates the attachments of the interosseous ligaments of the

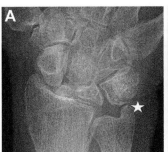
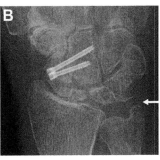

Fig. 11. Ulnar styloid triquetral impingement in a 45-year-old woman with KD with carpal collapse (*white star*). (*A*) Preoperative plain radiographs. (*B*) Postoperative radiographs following arthroscopic scaphocapitate fusion showing scaphoid extension, improvement of carpal height, and resolution of ulnar styloid-triquetral impingement (*white arrow*). (*Courtesy of* Simon MacLean, MBChB, FRCS(Tr&Orth), PGDipCE, North Island, New Zealand).

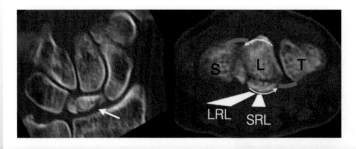

Fig. 12. Lunate ligament attachment fractures/attachments creating a spectrum of carpal instability. *Internal lunate instability* (*white arrow*), is instability due to fractures within the lunate, that lead to movement between the proximal and distal subchondral bone plates. *Intrinsic carpal instability* due to the avulsion of the lunate attachments to the dorsal scapholunate ligament and volar lunotriquetral ligaments (*yellow arrows*). *Extrinsic carpal instability* due to the coronal fracture involving the volar horn with the attached short and long radiolunate ligaments (SRL and LRL). S, scaphoid; L, lunate; T, triquetrum. (*Courtesy of* Greg Bain, PhD, MBBS, FRACS, FA(Ortho)A, Adelaide, Australia and Simon MacLean, MBChB, FRCS(Tr&Orth), PGDipCE, North Island, New Zealand).

lunate. The volar horn fragment of the lunate remains isometric with the stronger volar band of the lunotriquetral ligament, whereas the stronger dorsal band of the scapholunate ligament remains attached to the dorsal horn of the lunate. This leads to separation of these fragments in different wrist positions. Radiologically, this is shown as flattening and widening of the fractured lunate on loading and throughout different wrist positions.[8]

Ulnar Translocation

On reviewing dynamic motion of the KD wrist, we believe ulnar translocation can occur by 3 mechanisms:

1. *Attenuation* of extrinsic ligaments as a result of synovitis.
2. *Pseudo-laxity* of the extrinsic ligaments following central column collapse
3. *Direct avulsion* of the long and short radiolunate ligaments with the fragmented volar horn of the lunate.

As carpal height decreases and the capitate migrates proximally, the radioscaphocapitate ligament and dorsal radiocarpal ligaments develop

"pseudo-laxity," as ligament length remains isometric but carpal bone positions change. This leads to coronal instability. With compromise to the radioscaphocapitate and radiolunate ligaments, the carpus can translocate ulnar-wards. Taleisnik type-1 and type-2 ulnar translocation occurs, depending on the integrity of the scapholunate ligament. In all cases of ulnar translocation in our series, the lunate had a coronal fracture with associated avulsion of the attachments of the radiolunate ligaments[8] (**Fig. 13**). The management of ulnar translocation of the carpus is a challenging clinical problem. Certainly, in KD it should be identified when present. Surgical strategies used to revascularize, unload, or bypass the KD lunate should also take into consideration this pathology, as failure to manage translocation can lead to persistent symptoms and failure of the carpus.

CORRELATION WITH DISEASE PROGRESSION
Correlation of Degeneration with Dynamic Pathology

Lichtman and Bain[31] described progressive changes of collapse and degeneration in the Kienböck wrist. Bain and colleagues[28] described

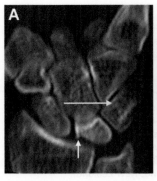
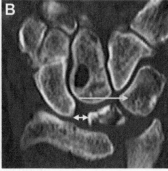

Fig. 13. Ulnar translocation. Coronal CT images Two types of ulnar translocation can be diagnosed in advanced stages of KD; Taleisnik type 1 (*A*) with avulsion-fracture of scapholunate ligament (*single-ended white arrow*), and type 2 (*B*) with associated scapholunate diastasis (*double-ended white arrow*). Note sclerosis at the scaphoid fossa in both cases and the scaphotrapeziotrapezoid (STT) degenerative changes in (*B*). (*Courtesy of* Simon MacLean, MBChB, FRCS(Tr&Orth), PGDipCE, North Island, New Zealand)

Correlation of Collapse with Dynamic Pathology

We have compared pathology diagnosed on dynamic 4D-CT imaging in patients with different stages of the disease. With advancing stage of the disease, more dynamic pathology is present. Effective surgical treatment of the patient with KD should take into account these pathologies (**Fig. 15**).

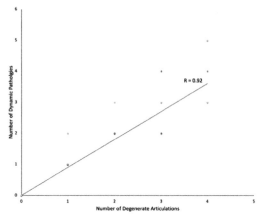

Fig. 14. Scatter plot showing number of dynamic pathologies identified on dynamic CT scanning versus the number of degenerate articulations. A regression line is shown with the gradient representing high correlation. (*Courtesy of* Simon MacLean, MBChB, FRCS(Tr&Orth), PGDipCE, North Island, New Zealand).

degenerative changes occurring at arthroscopy. There is a strong correlation between the number of degenerate articulations in the KD wrist and the presence of these dynamic pathologies. Although strongly associated, further studies are needed to imply any causation of these factors[8] (**Fig. 14**).

Correlation to Symptoms

Improved understanding of the disease pathology clearly improves our understanding of symptoms. Pain with KD has been generally regarded as central in the wrist as a result of synovitis, degeneration, and carpal collapse. Patients, however, may also report ulnar-sided pain and mechanical symptoms from ulnar styloid triquetral impingement. Volar pain and mechanical symptoms from volar radiolunate impingement can occur. Weakness and mechanical symptoms can result from dynamic instability in early stages of the disease, or ulnar translocation of the carpus in later stages. Pain correlation diagrams may aid the clinician to determine the site of pain in these cases.

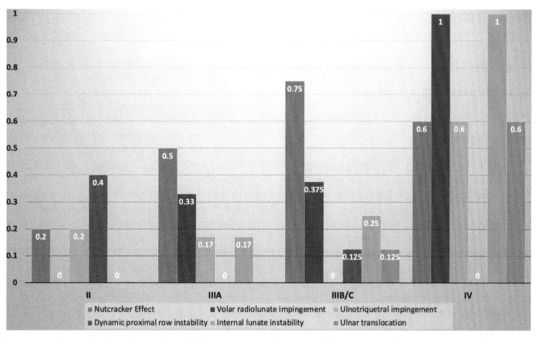

Fig. 15. Bar chart showing dynamic pathologies versus Lichtman grade. Figures on bars represent the finding as a proportion of patients at each Lichtman grade. (*Courtesy of* Simon MacLean, MBChB, FRCS(Tr&Orth), PGDipCE, North Island, New Zealand)

SUMMARY

Clearly, the etiology and pathogenesis of KD is multifactorial, leading to chondral, vascular, and osseous changes to both the lunate and the wrist. Through study of dynamic imaging, we now understand some of the important patho-mechanical aspects of the disease. It is likely that a "perfect storm" of biological and mechanical risk factors are required for the lunate to fail and for the disease to progress. Further prospective work on the kinematics of the disease should identify whether there is a defined dynamic "trigger" that affects the progression of the disease.

CLINICS CARE POINTS

- Radiographs and static CT identify osseous changes in KD. Chondral changes are best assessed with arthroscopy, and vascular status of the lunate with gadolinium-enhanced MRI. Dynamic pathology is best assessed with 4D-dynamic CT scanning.

- Symptomatology in KD is multifactorial, and may result from synovitis, instability, arthritis, and impingement.

- Surgical treatment should be tailored to each individual patient to address this complex range of pathology.

DISCLOSURE

The authors have nothing to disclose.

REFERENCES

1. Kienbock R. Concerning traumatic malacia of the lunate and its consequences: joint degeneration and compression. Fortsch Geb Roentgen 1910;16: 77–103.
2. Hultén O. Uber anatomische variationen der handgelenkknochen. Acta Radiol 1928;9(2):155–68.
3. Müller W. Über die Erweichung und Verdichtung des Os lunatum, eine typische Erkrankung des Handgelenks. Beitr Zur Klin Chir 1920;119:664.
4. Nakamura R, Tanaka Y, Imaeda T, et al. The influence of age and sex on ulnar variance. J Hand Surg Edinb Scotl 1991;16(1):84–8.
5. D'Hoore K, De Smet L, Verellen K, et al. Negative ulnar variance is not a risk factor for Kienböck's disease. J Hand Surg Am 1994;19(2):229–31.
6. Bain GI, MacLean SBM, Lichtman DM. Kienbock's Disease in Green's Hand Surgery. expertconsult.inkling.com
7. Bain GI, MacLean S, Yeo C, et al. The etiology and pathogenesis of Kienböck Disease. J Wrist Surg 2016;05(04):248–54.
8. MacLean SBM, Bain GI. Kinematics of the wrist in Kienböck's disease: a four-dimensional computed tomography study. J Hand Surg Eur 2021;46(5): 504–9.
9. MacLean SBM, Bain GI. Long-term outcome of surgical treatment for Kienböck disease using an articular-based classification. J Hand Surg Am 2021;46(5):386–95.
10. Rennie C, Britton J, Prouse P. Bilateral avascular necrosis of the lunate in a patient with severe Raynaud's phenomenon and scleroderma. J Clin Rheumatol Pract Rep Rheum Musculoskelet Dis 1999;5(3):165–8.
11. Lanzer W, Szabo R, Gelberman R. Avascular necrosis of the lunate and sickle cell anemia. A case report. Clin Orthop 1984;187:168–71.
12. Irisarri C. Aetiology of Kienbock's disease. J Hand Surg Am 2004;29(3):281–7.
13. Rooker GD, Goodfellow JW. Kienbock's disease in cerebral palsy. J Bone Jt Surg Br 1977;59(3):363–5.
14. Leclercq C, Xarchas C. Kienbock's disease in cerebral palsy. J Hand Surg Br 1998;23(6):746–8.
15. Culp RW, Schaffer JL, Osterman AL, et al. Kienböck's disease in a patient with Crohn's enteritis treated with corticosteroids. J Hand Surg Am 1989; 14(2 Pt 1):294–6.
16. Viegas SF, Wagner K, Patterson R, et al. Medial (hamate) facet of the lunate. J Hand Surg Am 1990;15(4):564–71.
17. Zapico J. Malacia del semilunar. Tesis doctoral. Universidad de Valladolid. Industrias y Editorial Sever Cuesta, Valladolid. In: Taleisnik J. The wrist. New York: Churchill Livingstone; 1985. p. 171–2.
18. Low SC, Bain GI, Findlay DM, et al. External and internal bone micro-architecture in normal and Kienböck's lunates: a whole-bone micro-computed tomography study. J Orthop Res 2014;32(6): 826–33.
19. Ueba Y, Kakinoki R, Nakajima Y, et al. Morphology and histology of the collapsed lunate in advanced Kienböck disease. Hand Surg Int J Devoted Hand Up Limb Surg Relat Res J Asia-pac Fed Soc Surg Hand 2013;18(2):141–9.
20. Lee ML. The intraosseus arterial pattern of the carpal lunate bone and its relation to avascular necrosis. Acta Orthop Scand 1963;33:43–55.
21. Gelberman R, Bauman T. The vascularity of the lunate bone and Kienböck's disease. J Hand Surg Am 1980;5(3):272–8.
22. Crock HV. An atlas of vascular anatomy of the skeleton & spinal cord. London, UK: Martin Dunitz; 1996.

23. Glueck CJ, Freiberg RWP. Heritable thrombophilia-hypofibrinolysis and osteonecrosis of the femoral head. Clin Orthop Relat Res 2008;466(5):1034–40.

24. Schiltenwolf M, Martini AK, Mau HC, et al. Further investigations of the intraosseous pressure characteristics in necrotic lunates (Kienböck's disease). J Hand Surg Am 1996;21(5):754–8.

25. Jensen CH. Intraosseous pressure in Kienböck's disease. J Hand Surg Am 1993;18(2):355–9.

26. Schmitt R, Heinze A, Fellner F, et al. Imaging and staging of avascular osteonecroses at the wrist and hand. Eur J Radiol 1997;25(2):92–103.

27. Bain GI, Durrant A. An articular-based approach to Kienbock avascular necrosis of the lunate. Tech Hand Up Extrem Surg 2011;15(1):41–7.

28. Bain G, MacLean S, Tse WL, et al. Kienböck disease and arthroscopy: assessment, classification, and treatment. J Wrist Surg 2016;05(04):255–60.

29. Lichtman DM, Mack GR, MacDonald RI, et al. Kienböck's disease: the role of silicone replacement arthroplasty. J Bone Joint Surg Am 1977;59(7): 899–908.

30. Topper SM, Wood MB, Ruby LK. Ulnar styloid impaction syndrome. J Hand Surg Am 1997;22(4): 699–704.

31. Lichtman DM, Bain GI. Kienbock's disease: advances in diagnosis and treatment. 1st edition. Springer; 2016.

Classification and Radiographic Characterization of Kienböck Disease

W. Charles Lockwood, MD[a,b], Alexander Lauder, MD[a,b],*

KEYWORDS

• Kienböck • Classification • Lichtman • Bain • Swanson • Nakamura • Schmitt

KEY POINTS

- The osseous classification of Kienböck disease is described by the Lichtman scheme, which categorizes the disease based on anticipated radiographic progression into 4 stages.
- Differentiating between Lichtman stage IIIA and IIIB is critical in treatment planning, and can be differentiated with a radioscaphoid angle of greater than 60°, indicating scaphoid flexion and carpal malalignment.
- MRI helps diagnose radiographically occult disease, and may be helpful to track lunate revascularization after intervention; gadolinium contrast may improve sensitivity and differentiate reversible ischemia from irreversible necrosis.
- The Bain and Begg arthroscopic classification scheme has been widely adopted as it guides treatment based upon the functional articulations surrounding the lunate.

INTRODUCTION

Robert Kienböck, a Viennese radiologist, first described radiographic changes associated with idiopathic lunate osteonecrosis in 1910 which he termed "traumatische Malazie" (traumatic malacia).[1] Since his first description, the radiographic progression of the condition that now bears his name has been well-described to progress from normal radiographs, to lunate sclerosis, followed by lunate collapse, proximal capitate migration, scaphoid flexion, and the ultimately the development of pancarpal arthritis.[2] Although the exact mechanism of Kienböck disease (KD) remains a topic of continued investigation, the anticipated progression of disease is better understood. Historically, a diagnosis correlating history, examination, and radiographic findings had been difficult in the early stages of the disease that did not manifest with obvious radiographic changes. As imaging modalities have evolved over the last century, diagnosis of the initial stages of the condition has become possible with MRI and may direct earlier treatment.

A thorough understanding of the progression of the disease is important in treating patients with the condition. Although numerous classification systems exist, the Lichtman classification, which describes the progression of degenerative changes seen on radiographs, and the Bain arthroscopic grading system, which defines the functional status of the intermediate column articular surfaces adjacent to the lunate, have become widely used[2,3]; the former for its description of the progression of the disease, and the latter because it guides treatment options and recommendations. An ideal classification system incorporates simplicity in understanding each stage of

a Department of Orthopedics, University of Colorado School of Medicine, 13001 E 17th Pl, Aurora, CO 80045, USA; b Department of Orthopedic Surgery, Denver Health Medical Center, 777 Bannock Street, Denver, CO 80207, USA
* Corresponding author.
E-mail address: Lauder.Alexander@gmail.com

Hand Clin 38 (2022) 405–415
https://doi.org/10.1016/j.hcl.2022.03.004

a condition, is highly reproducible between observers, and simultaneously can guide treatment. The treatment for KD can be broadly categorized as 1 of 5 types of intervention, including decompression, revascularization, unloading, reconstruction, or salvage.[4] Although a perfect classification system does not exist for KD, this article outlines the available classification systems and aims to highlight when each may be useful in the management of patients with this condition.

RADIOGRAPHIC CLASSIFICATION
Lichtman Classification

The Lichtman classification of KD describes the radiographic progression of the condition through 4 stages as diagnosed on plain radiographs of the wrist (**Figs. 1–2**, **Table 1**). This classification has been the mainstay for describing the severity of disease progression for multiple decades and has evolved since its origin, with the earliest documented version presented by Stahl in 1947.[5] It began as a 4-part radiographic classification describing the sequential stages of idiopathic avascular lunatomalacia. This system was later modified by Lichtman, who presented his version in 1977 within a case series of silicone lunate arthroplasties.[6] He concluded that treatment of the condition when it presents in earlier stages resulted in improved outcomes, and thus aimed to better define early and late disease. He used this information to inform his version of the 4-stage classification with the following goals: (1) to define a preoperative staging system that could guide appropriate treatment and (2) to use this staging system to allow for the retrospective comparison of outcomes based on various treatment to each stage of the disease. The stages of the Lichtman modification of the Stahl classification are provided in this article with descriptions of their specific findings and relevant adaptations over time.

Stage I
Plain radiographs of the lunate typically identify normal osseous architecture and lunate density with the diagnosis of KD suggested from clinical examination findings (**Fig. 2**A). Subtle radiographic abnormalities may show linear or compression

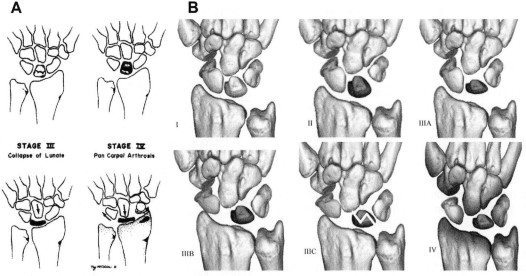

Fig. 1. Lichtman classification. (*A*) The original 4-stage Lichtman modification of the Stahl classification of KD. Stage I, normal radiographs or nondisplaced fracture lines. Stage II, density changes on plain radiographs. Stage III, lunate fragmentation, carpal collapse, with or without the "ring sign" of the flexed scaphoid. Stage IV, the addition radiographic evidence of perilunate arthrosis. (*B*) The modified/current 6-stage osseous radiographic Lichtman classification. Stage I, normal carpal alignment, often no plain radiographic evidence of boney changes. Stage II, sclerosis of lunate. Stage IIIA, maintained carpal alignment, lunate collapse, and fragmentation (radioscaphoid angle of <60°). Stage IIIB, lunate collapse and fragmentation with associated carpal collapse and scaphoid flexion (radioscaphoid angle of ≥60°). Stage IIIC, associated coronally oriented lunate fracture. Stage IV, evidence of advanced carpal collapse with perilunate carpal arthrosis. ([*A*] *From* Alexander AH, Turner MA, Alexander CE, Lichtman DM. Lunate silicone replacement arthroplasty in Kienböck's disease: a long-term follow-up. J Hand Surg Am. 1990 May;15(3):401-7;[8] with permission; and [*B*] Lichtman DM, Pientka WF 2nd, Bain GI. Kienböck Disease: A New Algorithm for the 21st Century. J Wrist Surg. 2017 Feb;6(1):2-10;[4] with permission.)

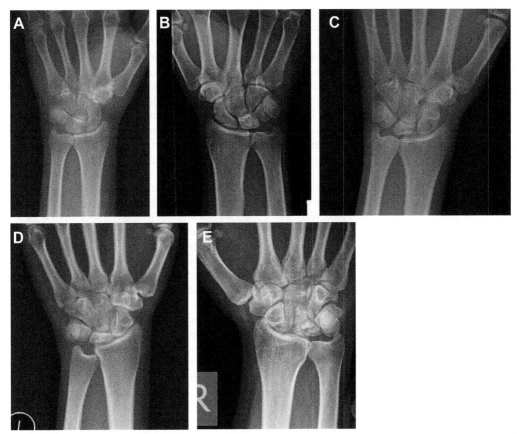

Fig. 2. Radiographic examples of the Lichtman stages. (*A*) Stage I, normal left wrist radiographs. (*B*) Stage II identifies lunate sclerosis. (*C*) Stage IIIA identified by lunate collapse without scaphoid flexion. (*D*) Stage IIIB shows lunate collapse with scaphoid flexion and the ring sign. (*E*) Stage IV with lunate collapse and pancarpal arthritic changes. (*Courtesy of* Alexander Lauder MD, Denver, CO.)

Table 1
Lichtman classification

Disease Stage	Radiographic Findings	MRI Findings	Treatment
I	Normal	T1 signal: decreased T2 signal: variable	Immobilization
II	Lunate sclerosis	T1 signal: decreased T2 signal: variable	Ulnar shortening (negative ulnar variance) Capitate Shortening (positive ulnar variance)
IIIA	Lunate collapse	T1 signal: decreased T2 signal: variable	Same as stage II, and/or Revascularization with dorsal pedicle
IIIB	Lunate and carpal collapse, Scaphoid rotation (RS angle of >60°)	T1 signal: decreased T2 signal: usually decreased	Reconstructive procedure STT or SC fusion ± lunate excision (if fragmented), or PRC
IV	Pancarpal arthritis KDAC	T1 signal: decreased T2 signal: decreased	Salvage procedure (TWF, TWA, or PRC)

Abbreviations: KDAC, Kienböck disease advanced collapse; PRC, proximal row carpectomy; RS, radioscaphoid; SC, scapho-capitate; TWA, total wrist arthroplasty; TWF, total wrist fusion.

From Lichtman DM, Pientka WF 2nd, Bain GI. Kienböck Disease: Moving Forward. J Hand Surg Am. 2016 May;41(5):630-8; with permission.

fractures of the lunate. In its original description, a bone scan was a useful diagnostic advanced imaging tool because it resulted in increased uptake in the lunate in patients with early KD not demonstrated on radiographs. With the improvement of MRI and its increased availability, MRI has replaced bone scan for early diagnosis of KD (stage I). MRI findings suggestive of KD include uniform decreased lunate signal intensity on both T1- and T2-weighted sequences representing marrow pathology associated with avascular necrosis.[2,7] Alternate findings may include decreased signal on T1 imaging with an increased T2 signal, indicating marrow edema.[2] The uniformity of the signal intensity pathognomonic for avascular necrosis is necessary to differentiate from ulnocarpal impaction, which has a treatment that is diametrically opposed to that of KD. The clinical symptoms in stage I may include pain that worsens with activity and improves with rest, often exacerbated by wrist extension and axial loading. Stage I KD is frequently misdiagnosed as a wrist sprain. Immobilization is the mainstay of treatment.

Stage II

The second stage is represented by radiodensity changes to the lunate. Sclerosis as well as lytic changes can be seen; however, the carpal architecture and intercarpal alignment remain unchanged (see **Fig. 2**B). Clinically, there can be increased swelling, night pain, and other symptoms consistent with synovitis. The treatment focus in stage II KD has historically consisted of lunate unloading or revascularization.

Stage III

Stage III KD is now subdivided into 2 substages based on the presence of lunate collapse with either normal scaphoid alignment (IIIA) or fixed scaphoid flexion (IIIB) (see **Fig. 2**C–D). Differentiating these substages is pivotal to guiding treatment. Clinically, patients experience pain with activity and at rest and can have progressive mechanical symptoms, including catching, locking, or grinding as disease severity increases.[1] In its original description, stage III, which did not initially have 2 subgroups, was defined as lunate collapse, proximal capitate migration, and disruption of the carpal architecture. In Lichtman's early case series, those in stage III KD often fared worse and had unpredictable surgical outcomes compared with other stages.[2] The outcome volatility prompted further analysis, which showed that lunate collapse and capitate migration did not happen simultaneously.[2] In 1982, Lichtman redefined and subdivided this stage into stages IIIA and IIIB.

Radiographically, stage IIIA reveals lunate fragmentation and collapse without changes in carpal alignment. Stage IIIB demonstrates lunate fragmentation and collapse with associated carpal malalignment, defined as rigid scaphoid flexion. Scaphoid flexion was originally identified by the presence of a scaphoid cortical ring sign seen on the posterior–anterior radiograph (see **Fig. 2**D). The ring sign represents the flexion of the distal pole of the scaphoid captured en face as it sits more perpendicular to the long axis of the radius. Stage IIIB, as the disease progresses, can also include proximal migration of the capitate representing carpal collapse.[8] The distinction between stages IIIA and IIIB is of great importance for treatment planning. Treatment of stages I through IIIA includes revascularization and lunate unloading via joint leveling procedures. However, once the carpal alignment shifts, as seen in stage IIIB KD, the associated carpal instability typically necessitates reconstruction or salvage procedures. Many clinicians have found the differentiation between stages IIIA and IIIB to be difficult.

Condit and colleagues[9] retrospectively analyzed 75 patients treated for KD over a 10-year period at a single institution. Their cohort was evaluated using a wrist outcome score assessing functional restrictions, range of motion deficits, and strength compared with the contralateral side. A score of poor was assigned if the patient went on to wrist arthrodesis. The authors analyzed changes in carpal alignment using the lunate index, carpal height index, ulnar negativity, scapholunate (SL) angle, and radioscaphoid (RS) angle. Regardless of treatment modality, the only measure that significantly correlated with outcome was the preoperative RS angle: a higher RS angle equating to worse outcome ($P < .001$) (**Fig. 3**). In the subgroup treated with joint leveling procedures, an RS angle of greater than 60° did not achieve either good or excellent outcomes.[9] The treatment algorithm at that time revolved around presence or absence of lunate collapse. These findings challenged that ideology and have helped to define the subgroups of stage III KD. Measuring the RS angle does not rely on the deformity of the lunate, but rather represents the presence of scaphoid flexion and carpal instability. The authors recommended using an RS angle of 60° as the threshold differentiating between Lichtman stages IIIA and IIIB.[9]

A concern regarding interobserver and intraobserver reliability in the Lichtman system led to an analysis of the reproducibility of the classification. In 1996, Jensen and colleagues[10] demonstrated poor reliability when 76 hand radiographs were examined by 2 orthopedic and 1 specialty trained hand surgeon with interobserver kappa values

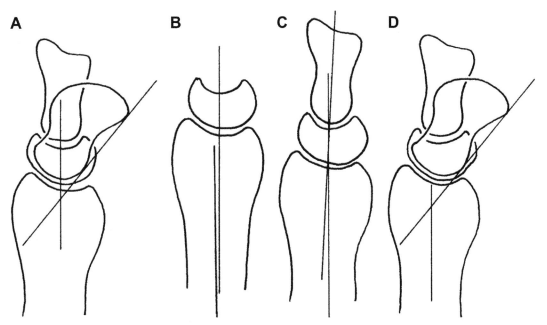

Fig. 3. Measurements of carpal alignment used in the assessment of KD. (*A*) Scapholunate angle. The scaphoid axis is represented by a line drawn tangent to the volar proximal and distal boundaries of the scaphoid. The lunate axis is represented by a line drawn perpendicular to a tangent connecting the volar and dorsal distal poles of the lunate. (*B*) Radiolunate angle. The line representing the radius is drawn through the center of the radius at 2 and 5 cm proximal to the joint. The lunate axis is represented by a line drawn perpendicular to a tangent connecting the volar and dorsal distal poles of the lunate. (*C*) Radiocapitate angle. The line representing the radius is drawn through the center of the radius at 2 and 5 cm proximal to the joint. The capitate is represented by a line through its proximal and distal poles (*D*) Radioscaphoid angle. The line representing the radius is drawn through the center of the radius at 2 and 5 cm proximal to the joint. The scaphoid line is drawn as a tangent to the volar proximal and distal boundaries of the scaphoid. An angle of 60° or greater, representing fixed flexion of the scaphoid differentiates Lichtman stage IIIA from IIIB. (*From* Goldfarb CA, Hsu J, Gelberman RH, Boyer MI. The Lichtman classification for Kienböck's disease: an assessment of reliability. J Hand Surg Am. 2003 Jan;28(1):74-80; with permission.)

between 0.45 and 0.52 and intraobserver kappa values between 0.26 and 0.63.[10] In 2000, Jafarnia and colleagues[11] published their assessment of Lichtman staging reliability investigating 4 surgeons, 3 of whom had completed a hand fellowship. The reviewers graded 74 radiographs and interobserver reliability showed a kappa value of 0.71 (range, 0.66–0.74), for all Lichtman stages combined; however, the authors did not publish a subanalysis of each stage of the Lichtman classification.[11]

Goldfarb and colleagues[12] evaluated the interobserver reliability specifically of Lichtman stages II, IIIA, and IIIB. Four surgeons with different levels of orthopedic training reviewed 39 patients. The films analyzed included posterior–anterior, lateral, and oblique radiographs for all individuals. They measured the SL angle, radiolunate angle, capitolunate angle, scaphocapitate angle, RS angle, carpal height, Stahl ratio, and the presence of a ring sign. Using the Lichtman classification, interobserver reliability of distinguishing IIIA from IIIB yielded a kappa value of 0.38 for IIIA and 0.62 for IIIB. When using an RS angle of greater than 60° as the differentiator between stage IIIA and IIIB, the kappa value increased to 0.75 for stage IIIA and 0.83 for IIIB, correlating with substantial and excellent agreement. Notably, the scaphoid ring sign did not correlate with other indicators of carpal collapse. These findings supported the previous results of Condit and colleagues[9] and reasoned that defining the Lichtman stage IIIB with an RS angle of greater than 60° was the best radiographic surrogate for scaphoid flexion and subsequent carpal collapse. Their investigation also showed that the other indices of SL angle, capitolunate, angle, carpal height ratio, and scaphoid cortical ring sign were not reliable in differentiation between stage IIIA and IIIB.[12] In 2010, Lichtman et al[2] proposed a class IIIC designation to the classification to include complete coronal plane fractures of the lunate and described poor healing potential of the IIIC lunate even after revascularization attempts, suggesting that salvage procedures involving lunate excision were needed.

Stage IV

Stage IV KD is defined as lunate collapse with associated degenerative arthritis of the radiocarpal and/or midcarpal joints (see **Fig. 2**E). Clinically, patients present with pain and stiffness consistent with advanced degenerative arthritis. Radiographically, the arthritic changes present are often very similar to the advanced collapse seen in SL advanced collapse or scaphoid non-union advanced collapse. For purposes of comparison, stage IV has also been termed KD advanced collapse.[2]

Stage 0 (conceptual)

The latest evolution of Lichtman's classification suggests the usefulness of adding stage 0 to identify and treat the patient without radiographic or MRI findings of KD but who may present with exertional ischemic pain.[2] Although the early diagnosis of patients with KD in this stage may afford earlier treatment, this stage has not had widespread adoption.

Swanson Classification

The Swanson classification (**Table 2**) uses radiographs to divide KD into a 6-stage progression in attempt to outline disease severity, similar to the Lichtman scheme. In 1985, Swanson and colleagues[13] retrospectively reviewed 42 cases of silicone arthroplasty implantation for patients with KD. Using the severity of bony changes in the lunate and surrounding carpal bones along with scaphoid rotation, carpal collapse, and carpal translation, the 6-stage classification was developed describing radiographic findings and associated treatment options. The 6 stages of the Swanson classification correlate with an augmented description of the disease progression corresponding to the analogous Lichtman stages II through IV. Their retrospective review highlighted the correlation between worsening lunate avascular necrosis and collapse in carpal height, increasing RS angle, and ulnar migration of the capitate.[13] This classification has not become widespread owing to its association with silicone arthroplasty, a procedure abandoned owing to high complication rates and failures; however, Swanson's use of the RS angle to helped inform the work of Lichtman, Condit, Goldfarb, and others.

MAGNETIC RESONANCE IMAGING CLASSIFICATION

Nakamura Classification

With the improvements in the accessibility and usability of MRI, multiple classifications emerged with MRI as the diagnostic test of choice. In 1993, Tsuge and Nakamura[14] reviewed 24 patients with KD (1 Lichtman I, 9 Lichtman II, 8 Lichtman III, 6 Lichtman IV) to investigate the effects of radial shortening versus radial wedge osteotomy. Preoperative and postoperative MRIs were obtained in all patients to examine lunate healing and revascularization. A 5-stage grading system was created assessing lunate signal intensity from both T1- and T2-weighted images (**Table 3**). The study identified an increase in the signal intensity in 18 of 19 patients undergoing radial osteotomy 1 year postoperatively. Interestingly, a subset showed improvement in T2 signal only, and overall T2 images had earlier signal intensity return compared with T1 imaging, indicating that T2-weighted images are more sensitive to lunate vascular changes.[14] These findings were corroborated by the work of other investigators, who also concluded that signal intensity increases with lunate healing.[15,16] This classification has not been adopted widely because it does not guide treatment for each progressive stage; however, the work helped to inform the diagnostic and prognostic use of MRI in KD. Additionally, the system does not require the use of intravenous gadolinium contrast and may allow for an assessment of lunate revascularization after a surgical intervention.

Schmitt Classification

A summary of the 3-stage Schmitt classification and specific enhancement of geographic areas of the lunate with T1-weighted, T2-weighted, and contrast-enhanced T1-weighted images is displayed in **Table 4**. Schmitt and colleagues[17] evaluated the lunate changes with contrast enhancement to the MRI. The study suggested that gadopentetate contrast in the presence of intact perfusion enhances interosseous signal intensity on T1-weighted imaging. Pathoanatomic characterization defined ischemia into 3 predictable zones: (1) the zone of necrosis, often at the proximal pole of the lunate without enhancement; (2) the intermediate hypervascular zone of repair with microscopic elements of recycling and reparation; and (3) the normal zone of viability often at the distal pole with intact perfusion. After evaluating the MRI images of 28 patients with KD, 3 distinct stages of ischemia were evident ranging from (A) edema with intact perfusion to (B) partially necrotic based on perfusion zone (proximal, middle, or distal), and finally (C) necrotic with poor viability. The authors noted that evaluation can be complicated in longstanding KD, which can create an enhancing synovitic reaction after

Table 2
Swanson classification for avascular necrosis of the lunate and treatments

Stage	Pathologic Findings	Treatments
I	Sclerosis of the lunate with minimal symptoms and normal carpal bone relationships	Splinting and rest, revascularization, and ulnar and radial lengthening or shortening
II	Sclerosis of the lunate with cystic changes with clinical symptoms and normal carpal bone relationships	Lunate implant replacement and ulnar and radial lengthening or shortening
III	Sclerosis, cysts, and fragmentation of the lunate with a scaphoid–radial angle 40–60°, carpal height collapse of 0%–5%, and carpal translation minimal	Lunate implant replacement with or without intercarpal fusions
IV	Sclerosis, cysts, and fragmentation of lunate with scaphoid–radial angle of <70°, carpal height collapse of 5%–10%, and carpal translation moderate	Lunate implant replacement with scaphoid stabilization (distal fusion) and intercarpal fusion if early changes in contiguous bones
V	Sclerosis, cysts, and fragmentation of lunate, with a scaphoid radial angle of >70°, carpal height collapse of >10%, sever carpal translation, and cystic changes in contiguous bones	Lunate implant replacement and intercarpal fusion, scapholunate implant replacement, wrist arthrodesis, and ulna impingement treatment as needed
VI	Sclerosis, cysts, and fragmentation of lunate with a scaphoid radial angle of >70°, carpal height collapse of >15%, sever carpal translation, cystic changes in contiguous bones, and significant intercarpal and radiocarpal degenerative arthritic changes	Total wrist implant arthroplasty, wrist arthrodesis, and ulnar impingement treatment as needed

The 6-stage Swanson descriptive classification of pathologic findings associated with idiopathic avascular necrosis of the lunate, and associated treatments. This classification is no longer used as the implant arthroplasty was associated with predictable catastrophic failures, yet the adjunctive other treatments are still used today.
From Swanson AB, Maupin BK, de Groot Swanson G, Ganzhorn RW, Moss SH. Lunate implant resection arthroplasty: long-term results. J Hand Surg Am. 1985 Nov;10(6 Pt 2):1013-24; with permission.

Table 3
Nakamura MRI grading system for KD

Grade	Coronal T1- or T2-Weighted MRI Findings
I	Normal (isointensity)
II	Localized regions of slightly decreased signal intensity
III	Generalized slight decrease in signal intensity
IV	Low signal intensity with regions of high or isointensity signals
V	Generalized low signal intensity

From Matsui Y, Funakoshi T, Motomiya M, Urita A, Minami M, Iwasaki N. Radial shortening osteotomy for Kienböck disease: minimum 10-year follow-up. J Hand Surg Am. 2014 Apr;39(4):679-85; with permission.

application of contrast.[18] The addition of contrast was found to be most useful in the differentiation of intercellular (reversible) edema and intracellular (irreversible) edema. Without contrast, the T2-weighted sequence signal height was similar in necrotic, reparative, and normal bone marrow.[17] Additionally, T1 sequences were found to overestimate osteonecrosis, because both reparation and necrosis may be isointense. The use of gadolinium contrast may improve sensitivity and differentiate reversible ischemia from irreversible necrosis.[19] Although the Schmitt classification characterizes the lunate in significant detail, the classification scheme does not guide clinical management for KD.

ARTHROSCOPIC CLASSIFICATION
Bain and Begg Classification

The arthroscopic Bain and Begg grading system describes the functional status of the intermediate

Table 4
Schmitt classification of lunate vascularity/viability

Pattern	MRI Findings	Prognosis
N	Normal signal	NA
A	Homogeneous enhancement of lunate with marrow edema; *intact lunate perfusion*	Good
B	Inhomogeneous signal with enhancement of the reparative zone and viable distal bone; necrotic proximal lunate (*partial osteonecrosis*)	Intermediate
C	No contrast enhancement; *complete osteonecrosis*	Poor

The Schmitt classification can be broadly summarized into 4 categories: (N) normal, (A) ischemic, (B) partially necrotic based on perfusion zone (proximal middle, or distal), and (C) necrotic with poor viability.
From Lichtman DM, Pientka WF 2nd, Bain GI. Kienböck Disease: Moving Forward. J Hand Surg Am. 2016 May;41(5):630-8; with permission.

column articular surfaces adjacent to the lunate (**Fig. 4**).[3] KD typically develops initially with arthritic changes of the proximal articular surface of the lunate with secondary changes to the lunate facet of the distal radius. As arthritis progresses in KD, the distal surface of the lunate and finally proximal portion of the capitate become involved. As such, the Bain and Begg 5-stage grading system mirrors this progression of articular degeneration while also aiming to guide surgical treatment based on the number of nonfunctional articular surfaces. In 2006, Bain and Begg described their approach using arthroscopy to assess and classify KD. In their description, wrist arthroscopy performed in a standard fashion allows identification of synovitis and assessment of the articular surfaces adjacent to the lunate. The authors surmised that arthroscopy both provides a diagnostic tool and directs definitive surgery based on the intraoperative findings. When articular surfaces are deemed functional, synovectomy, decompression, revascularization, or unloading procedures may be performed.[3] When articular surfaces are nonfunctional, defined

as having extensive fibrillation, fissuring, articular loss, or fracture, reconstruction or salvage procedures such as proximal row carpectomy, radioscapholunate arthrodesis, or wrist arthrodesis may be performed, depending on the extent of joint involvement. This classification scheme has been well-adopted because it mirrors the progressive development of arthritis in addition to providing treatment options at each stage. Additionally, advanced imaging such as MRI or computed tomography (CT) scans can be used in lieu of arthroscopy to determine the status of the articular surfaces.

COMBINED CLASSIFICATION

In 2017, a collaboration of multiple classifications schemes to better inform diagnosis and treatment was developed (**Fig. 5**).[4] Considering the patient's age, lunate revascularization potential, and individual carpal pathoanatomic characteristics, the combined classification simplified the many useful schemes. Lichtman and Bain separated the algorithm into 3 sections: (A) age, (B) stage of the lunate, and (C) state of the wrist. Section (A) divides patient age into 3 subgroups with potential for good success of nonoperative treatment: less than 15 years of age, 16 to 20 years of age, and more than 70 years of age. Patients between the ages of 21 and 70 were then analyzed separately in sections (B) and (C) with operative considerations. Section (B) is subdivided into 3 parts evaluating lunate integrity with associated treatment suggestions. Section (C) is split up into 4 subgroups based on the amount of articular compromise and carpal collapse.[4]

COMPUTED TOMOGRAPHY SCANS

Plain radiographs typically underestimate the extent of the disease process compared with CT scans.[20] Advanced imaging with CT scans aids in the understanding of osseous sclerosis, fragmentation, collapse, and adjacent articular arthritis and is helpful in surgical planning.[21] Although there are no classification systems specific to the use of CT imaging, the aforementioned classifications can be diagnosed more precisely with the use of CT scans and should be considered for all patients with KD.

DISCUSSION

As imaging modalities have advanced and evolved, so have the classifications systems describing KD. The 4-stage Stahl classification progressed into the modified 6-stage Lichtman classification, which remains a commonly used

Grade	Description	Recommendation
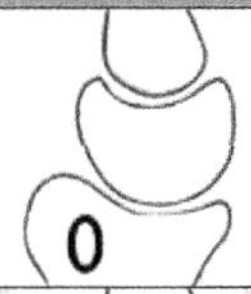 0	**Grade 0** 0 Nonfunctional surface	Joint levelling procedure Forage ± bone graft Vascularized bone graft
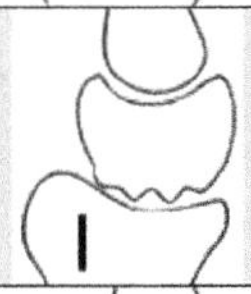 1	**Grade 1** 1 Nonfunctional surface - Proximal lunate	RSL fusion PRC Osteochondral grafting
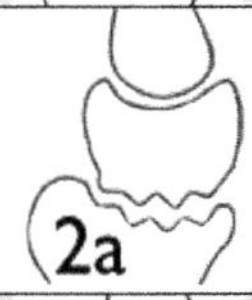 2a	**Grade 2a** 2 Nonfunctional surfaces - Proximal lunate and lunate facet of radius	RSL fusion
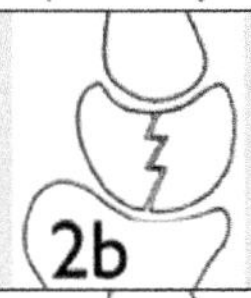 2b	**Grade 2b** 2 Nonfunctional surfaces - Proximal and distal lunate	PRC Lunate replacement Capitate Lengthening
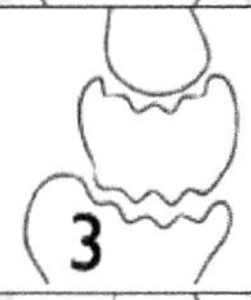 3	**Grade 3** 3 Nonfunctional surfaces - Capitate surface usually preserved	Hemiarthroplasty (SC fusion if radial column intact)
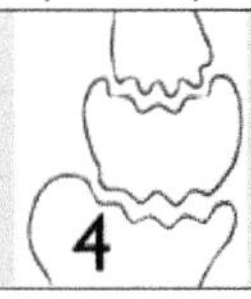 4	**Grade 4** All 4 articular surfaces are nonfunctional	Total wrist fusion Total wrist arthroplasty (SC fusion if radial column intact)

Synovectomy is performed in all patients.

PRC, proximal row carpectomy; RSL fusion, radioscapholunate fusion; SC fusion, scaphocapitate fusion; can be considered if the central column is nonfunctional, but the radial column is intact.

Fig. 4. Bain and Begg arthroscopic classification of KD. The grade is determined by the number of nonfunctional articular surfaces, originally based on arthroscopic assessment. The grading system assists the surgeon to determine the best surgical treatment, based on pathologic findings. (*From* Lichtman DM, Pientka WF 2nd, Bain GI. Kienböck Disease: Moving Forward. J Hand Surg Am. 2016 May;41(5):630-8; and Bain GI, Begg M. Arthroscopic assessment and classification of Kienbock's disease. Tech Hand Up Extrem Surg. 2006 Mar;10(1):8-13; with permissions.)

staging system and is often considered when planning treatment. Originally, Lichtman and associates[2] used radiographs to differentiate pathology and guide treatment. MRI has since been shown to help diagnose stage I disease with evidence of lunate edema.[14] Carpal kinematics and RS angular measurements have been integrated to differentiate stage IIIA from IIIB, defining an RS angle of more than 60° to indicate carpal instability with significant scaphoid flexion.[9] High-resolution CT scanning has become valuable to identify early stage II lytic changes, early stage IIIA fragmentation, nondisplaced stage IIIC fractures, and early perilunate osteoarthritis of stage IV; however, the use of CT scans frequently result in upstaging the disease.[20] The addition of contrast-enhanced MRI has added elements of prognosis allowing for differentiation between irreversible necrosis and reversible cellular injury. MRI may be helpful in determining revascularization of the lunate after interventions.[14,18] The diagnostic use of arthroscopy in determining functional articulating surfaces abutting the lunate has allowed for the development of a classification system that easily guides treatment options and overall follows the evolution of the disease. Currently, an all-encompassing imaging classification that both guides treatment and prognosis does not exist.

A. Patient's age?

　　A1. < 15 y – Non-operative

　　A2. 16 –20 y – Non-operative first. Consider unloading procedure.

　　A3. > 70 years – Non-operative first. Consider synovectomy and / or follow algorithm below.

B. Stage of the lunate?

　　B1. Lunate intact (Cortex and cartilage intact – Lichtman 0, I, II, Schmitt A, Bain 0)

　　Protect / unload the lunate:

　　Orthosis or cast first (trial for 2–3 months)

　　Radial shortening osteotomy, capitate shortening for ulnar +ve (radial epiphysiodesis[a])

　　(Alternatives – Lunate decompression, vascularized bone graft[a], radius forage[a])

　　B2. Lunate compromised (Localized lunate disease – Lichtman IIIA, Schmitt B, Bain 1)

　　Lunate reconstruction: MFT[a], lunate replacement[a], PRC (RSL fusion, SC [or STT] fusion)

　　B3. Lunate not reconstructable (Advanced lunate disease - Lichtman IIIC, Schmitt C, Bain 2b)

　　Lunate salvage (excision): Lunate replacement[a], capitate lengthening, PRC (SC fusion)

C. State of the wrist?

　　C1. Central column articulations compromised (Lichtman IIIA or C, Schmitt B, Bain 2a, 3, or 4)

　　　　C1a. Radiolunate articulation compromised (Lichtman IIIA, Schmitt B, Bain 2a)

　　　　Fuse or Bypass radiolunate joint: RSL fusion, SC fusion, Lunate Prosthesis, MFT graft

　　　　C1b. Radiolunate and midcarpal articulations compromised (Lichtman IIIA or C, Schmitt B, Bain 3 or 4)

　　　　Bypass central column: SC fusion

　　C2. Carpal collapse with intact radioscaphoid articulation (Lichtman IIIB or C, Schmitt B, Bain 2 - 4)

　　Stabilize radial column: SC fusion

　　C3. Wrist not reconstructable (Advanced wrist disease – Lichtman IV, Schmitt C, Bain 4)

　　Wrist salvage: Total wrist arthrodesis, total wrist arthroplasty[a]

Other options that can be considered have been placed in (parentheses). STT fusion is an alternative to SC fusion.
[a]Alternate procedures, techniques that require specialized skills and therefore affect what the surgeon can offer.
The classification determines the recommended treatment based on the patient's age (A), status of the lunate (B) and the status of the wrist (C).
What the surgeon can offer (D) and what the patient wants (E) ultimately determine what is performed.

Fig. 5. The key questions for KD: a new algorithm. The most recent classification and algorithm combines prior schemes incorporating patient age, radiographic, MRI, and arthroscopic findings. (*From* Lichtman DM, Pientka WF 2nd, Bain GI. Kienböck Disease: A New Algorithm for the 21st Century. J Wrist Surg. 2017 Feb;6(1):2-10; with permission.)

However, a current clinical assessment of lunatomalacia to include modified Lichtman staging and Bain arthroscopic grading, as well as Schmitt ischemia staging using contrast-enhanced MRI gives great value in prognostication and management decisions.[4]

SUMMARY

Although much remains unclear regarding the optimal treatment for each of the various stages of KD progression, the available classification schemes are helpful in predicting disease progression, allow for a comprehensive understanding of relevant pathology, and guide management for patients with KD.

CLINICS CARE POINTS

- The radiographic progression of KD advances from normal radiographs, to lunate sclerosis, lunate collapse, proximal capitate migration, scaphoid flexion, and the ultimate development of pancarpal arthritis.[2]

- The treatment for KD can be broadly categorized as 1 of 5 types of intervention, including decompression, revascularization, unloading, reconstruction, or salvage.[4]

- Advanced imaging modalities have evolved over time to allow the diagnosis of early stages of KD when radiographs are nondiagnostic.

- The radiographic osseous classification of KD based on the Lichtman scheme incorporates a 4-stage system that categorizes the disease based on anticipated radiographic progression.[2] Differentiating between stage IIIA and IIIB KD is critical in treatment concept, and can be distinguished by an RS angle of greater than 60°, representing fixed scaphoid flexion and carpal malalignment.

- The MRI classification schemes of Tsuge and Nakamura[14] and Schmitt and associates,[18,19] help to diagnose early stages of the disease when radiographs do not identify pathology, and MRI may identify lunate revascularization after interventions.

- The arthroscopic grading system described by Bain and Begg outlines the functional status of the intermediate column articular surfaces adjacent to the lunate and guides treatment options based on intraoperative findings.[3] This grading concept has been well accepted an can be extrapolated to treatment concepts inferred from imaging such as CT scans.

DISCLOSURE

The authors hold no conflicts of interest with the content presented within the manuscript.

REFERENCES

1. Kennedy C, Abrams R. In brief: the Lichtman classification for Kienbock disease. Clin orthopaedics Relat Res 2019;477(6):1516–20.
2. Lichtman DM, Lesley NE, Simmons SP. The classification and treatment of Kienbock's disease: the state of the art and a look at the future. J Hand Surg Eur volume 2010;35(7):549–54.
3. Bain GI, Begg M. Arthroscopic assessment and classification of Kienbock's disease. Tech Hand upper extremity Surg 2006;10(1):8–13.
4. Lichtman DM, Pientka WF 2nd, Bain GI. Kienbock Disease: a new algorithm for the 21st century. J Wrist Surg 2017;6(1):2–10.
5. Stahl F. On lunatomalacia (Kienböck's Disease). A clinical and roentgenological study, especially on its pathogenesis and the late results of immobilization treatment. Acta Chir Scand 1947;126(suppl): 1–133.
6. Lichtman DM, Mack GR, MacDonald RI, et al. Kienbock's disease: the role of silicone replacement arthroplasty. J bone Jt Surg Am volume 1977; 59(7):899–908.
7. Luo J, Diao E. Kienbock's disease: an approach to treatment. Hand Clin 2006;22(4):465–73.
8. Alexander AH, Turner MA, Alexander CE, et al. Lunate silicone replacement arthroplasty in Kienbock's disease: a long-term follow-up. J Hand Surg 1990;15(3):401–7.
9. Condit DP, Idler RS, Fischer TJ, et al. Preoperative factors and outcome after lunate decompression for Kienbock's disease. J Hand Surg 1993;18(4): 691–6.
10. Jensen CH, Thomsen K, Holst-Nielsen F. Radiographic staging of Kienbock's disease. Poor reproducibility of Stahl's and Lichtman's staging systems. Acta Orthop Scand 1996;67(3):274–6.
11. Jafarnia K, Collins ED, Kohl HW 3rd, et al. Reliability of the Lichtman classification of Kienbock's disease. J Hand Surg 2000;25(3):529–34.
12. Goldfarb CA, Hsu J, Gelberman RH, et al. The Lichtman classification for Kienbock's disease: an assessment of reliability. J Hand Surg 2003;28(1): 74–80.
13. Swanson AB, Maupin BK, de Groot Swanson G, et al. Lunate implant resection arthroplasty: long-term results. J Hand Surg 1985;10(6 Pt 2):1013–24.
14. Tsuge S, Nakamura R. Anatomical risk factors for Kienbock's disease. J Hand Surg 1993;18(1):70–5.
15. Sowa DT, Holder LE, Patt PG, et al. Application of magnetic resonance imaging to ischemic necrosis of the lunate. J Hand Surg 1989;14(6):1008–16.
16. Viegas SF, Amparo E. Magnetic resonance imaging in the assessment of revascularization in Kienbock's disease. A preliminary report. Orthop Rev 1989; 18(12):1285–8.
17. Schmitt R, Christopoulos G, Wagner M, et al. Avascular necrosis (AVN) of the proximal fragment in scaphoid nonunion: is intravenous contrast agent necessary in MRI? Eur J Radiol 2011;77(2):222–7.
18. Schmitt R, Heinze A, Fellner F, et al. Imaging and staging of avascular osteonecroses at the wrist and hand. Eur J Radiol 1997;25(2):92–103.
19. Schmitt R, Kalb K. Advanced Imaging of Kienböck's Disease. In: Kienböck's disease: advances in diagnosis and treatment. Springer; 2016.
20. Quenzer DE, Linscheid RL, Vidal MA, et al. Trispiral tomographic staging of Kienbock's disease. J Hand Surg 1997;22(3):396–403.
21. Schmitt R, Kalb K. [Imaging in Kienbock's Disease]. Handchir Mikrochir Plast Chir 2010;42(3):162–70. Bildgebende Diagnostik der Lunatumnekrose.

An Algorithmic Approach to the Treatment of Kienböck Disease

Joseph Catapano, MD, PhD[a], James P. Higgins, MD[b],*

KEYWORDS

- Avascular necrosis • Kienböck disease • Lunate

KEY POINTS

- Kienböck disease is associated with several factors that predispose the lunate to avascular necrosis and collapse.
- Management of Kienböck disease is assessed in the context of each individual patient presentation.
- Broad treatment categories address lunate unloading, lunate revascularization, and ablation.
- Surgical algorithms can be devised based on a combination of established staging systems.

INTRODUCTION

Compared with many challenging problems in hand surgery, Kienböck disease has a plethora of variables that may impact the evolution of a surgeon's treatment algorithm: etiology continues to be debated, the rate of progression is unknown, and proposed treatments are numerous and supported by inconsistent literature. The incidence of disease is low and the complexity and required skillset for various interventions varies widely, limiting the breadth of experience of individual surgeons. Kienböck disease also presents in a younger demographic with high expectations of functional outcomes and minimal acceptance of arthritis, making common wrist operations used for other carpal problems, such as proximal row carpectomy and wrist fusion, less acceptable.

In this setting, surgeons will find a wide variety of recommendations with no distinct algorithm prescribed in the literature. Some of the greatest contributors to this body of literature are included in this text, contributing chapters on the foundation of our understanding of possible etiology, as well as the techniques for treatment and their respective outcomes. This installment is aimed at providing our algorithm for the treatment of this challenging disorder. Other surgeons have provided alternative approaches for various reasons. Herein we try to provide an explanation for the clinical factors we consider in making treatment decisions for the variety of presentations of Kienböck disease. Although algorithms for this process are often grouped according to a staging system, we first review the broad categories of treatment options, highlighting their benefits and drawbacks.

TREATMENT OPTIONS

Although the initiating pathologic event in Kienböck disease remains unknown, it is now recognized to occur in the "at-risk" patient predisposed to avascular necrosis of the lunate due to several contributory risk factors.[1] These include arterial supply,[2–4] venous hypertension,[5,6] ulnar negative variance,[7–11] radial inclination,[12,13] and lunate morphology. Although outside the scope of this publication, a detailed review of etiology can be reviewed elsewhere.[1,14]

[a] Division of Plastic and Reconstructive Surgery, St. Michael's Hospital, University of Toronto, 30 Bond Street, Donnelly Wing, Room 4-072, Toronto, ON M5B 1W8, Canada; [b] The Curtis National Hand Center, MedStar Union Memorial Hospital, 3333 North Calvert Street, JPB #200, Baltimore, MD 21218, USA
* Corresponding author.
E-mail address: editor@curtishand.com

Hand Clin 38 (2022) 417–424
https://doi.org/10.1016/j.hcl.2022.03.005

Surgical treatments for Kienböck disease address the perceived etiologic factors and can be broadly classified into (1) offloading, (2) revascularization, or (3) salvage procedures.

Immobilization

Nonoperative management remains a common treatment strategy early in the course of disease. A recent study of American Society for Surgery of the Hand (ASSH) members identified that 74% of surgeons manage Lichtman stage 1 disease with cast immobilization for an average of 7 weeks; this number reduced to 37% for stage 2.[15] Immobilization is particularly effective in the pediatric population, where progression to more advanced disease is less predictable.[16] Although few pediatric cases have been described in the literature, Irisarri and colleagues[17] described excellent outcomes with splinting in patients ages 12 or younger, in contrast to older pediatric patients in whom 30% progressed and required joint leveling. Similar results in pediatric patients with nonoperative management have been demonstrated by others.[18–20] Elderly patients also may respond well to conservative treatment with splinting to manage pain and permit activities of daily living. However, in contrast to pediatric patients, elderly patients tend to progress to carpal collapse despite excellent clinical outcomes with nonoperative management.[21,22]

In contrast to pediatric patients, the lunate in Kienböck disease presenting in skeletally mature, high-demand patients does not show the remodeling potential demonstrated in pediatric patients. Well documented by Kristensen and colleagues,[20] Mikkelsen and colleagues,[23] and Viljakka and colleagues,[24] although nonoperative management with splinting may be effective for pain management, it is frequently ineffective at preventing progression of disease to radiocarpal arthritis.

Our team includes a discussion of immobilization with all patients presenting with Kienböck disease. We present the option as unlikely to halt progression of the disease in adults. Thus, the option for immobilization is usually selected among 3 groups: (1) young teenagers with early-stage Kienböck disease, particularly when parents are interested in exhausting nonsurgical options; (2) patients older than 60 years, when the progression of disease may more readily be treated with ablative procedures, such as a proximal row carpectomy (PRC); and (3) the risk-averse patients requesting a trial of nonoperative management. To give immobilization an adequate opportunity to demonstrate effectiveness, we use 12 weeks of short arm casting. Thereafter, patients are monitored for persistent or worsening symptoms as they return to activities.

Unloading Procedures

Unloading procedures remain the most commonly performed procedures among ASSH members.[15] These procedures have the appeal of simplicity of technique, logical nature of treatment goals, and low morbidity of intervention. The 2 most widely used techniques, radial shortening osteotomy and capitate shortening osteotomy, are also supported by good biomechanical and clinical data.

Werner and colleagues[25] demonstrated that lengthening of the ulna by 2.5 mm increased the forces borne by the ulna from 18.4% to 41.9% of the total axial load, and likewise increasing the ulnocarpal load from 1.4 to 3.3 N/mm^2, suggesting that correcting ulnar variance can significantly alter wrist biomechanics. Trumble and colleagues[26] added to this by demonstrating that 2 mm of length change maximized lunate decompression without risking distal radioulnar joint or ulnocarpal impingement.

Radial shortening osteotomy (RSO) has demonstrated improved outcomes in comparison with nonoperative management in short-term follow-up in patients with stage 2 or 3 disease, demonstrating less pain and improved grip strength.[27] Although RSO has failed to reverse or prevent carpal collapse, patients report improved pain and slowed progression of radiologic disease. Several studies have reported on the efficacy of RSO in both short-term[27–31] and long-term studies.[24,32–37] Most studies report that changes in carpal height ratio and Stahl index remain stable; however, the arthritic disease tends to progress. Several investigators have reported good clinical outcomes using RSO for Kienböck disease, demonstrating good resolution of pain, maintenance of range of motion, and infrequent progression of disease requiring reoperation (13%–19%).[38–40]

In the context of ulnar neutral or ulnar positive variance, capitate shortening osteotomy (CSO) provides an excellent means of unloading the lunate. CSO has been hypothesized in mathematical models to decrease the radiolunate force by 66%, with axial forces on the wrist increasing the ulnar-triquetral force instead.[41] Offloading of the lunate has been confirmed in biomechanical studies as well.[42,43] Almquist[44] described immediate pain relief in patients undergoing CSO, hypothesizing that this was due to decreased forces across the lunate, relief of synovitis, and possibly due to denervation of the wrist during surgery.

In a retrospective comparison of 21 patients undergoing RSO (n = 12) or CSO (n = 9), following an average follow-up of 3 years, patients demonstrated no difference in pain visual analog scale (VAS) scores, range of motion, grip strength, or Disabilities of the Arm, Shoulder, and Hand (DASH) score.[45] All patients had stage 3A Kienböck disease and treatment was based on the presence of negative ulnar variance.[46] In 9 patients with stage 1 to stage 3A disease, capitate shortening osteotomy has been shown to improve vascularity of the lunate with MRI.[47] In a study investigating 17 patients with stage 2 or 3A disease, CSO demonstrated an improvement in pain scores (VAS 7.12–1.41), grip strength (47.12% to 75%), and wrist function scores.[48] Similar results were obtained in other studies.[46]

We consider these options in patients who demonstrate little or minimal collapse of the lunate. RSO is offered to ulnar negative patients and CSO is offered to ulnar neutral or ulnar positive patients. Although RSO has the significant advantage of being an extra-articular procedure, we have found minimal morbidity with CSO. With CSO, the capitate may be approached without releasing the extensor retinaculum. The radiocarpal capsule is not opened and a midcarpal osteotomy alone is required. After meticulous resection of 3 mm of the capitate, waist fixation may be achieved using longitudinal antegrade or oblique retrograde screws, or dorsal compression staples. We prefer the latter for its ease of application entirely away from the cartilage-bearing capitate head. Although both of these techniques show rapid and reliable osteotomy healing, we prefer to immobilize the wrist for 12 weeks following surgery in an attempt to garner the purported benefits of immobilization alongside the operative unloading.

Revascularization

Improving vascularization of the lunate is pursued using 3 different techniques: (1) drilling and core decompression, (2) vascularized bone flaps or blood vessels to revascularize the surrounding lunate shell, or (3) osteochondral flaps to replace most of the diseased lunate.

Drilling (of the radius, ulna, or lunate itself) with metaphyseal core decompression is thought to create an inflammatory response that may improve regional vascularity to the lunate. The procedure was first proposed by Illarramendi and colleagues[49] after experiencing the resolution of radiographic evidence of Kienböck disease in a patient with a nondisplaced distal radius fracture. Metaphyseal core decompression, typically performed in the dorsal radial metaphysis, presents a low-morbidity option as an extra-articular procedure. Although core decompression has demonstrated favorable results in the context of early disease, a limited number of studies have been published regarding outcomes and a physiologic explanation for the outcomes is lacking. Sherman and colleagues[50] investigated the biomechanical effect of core decompression of the distal radius, and found that although decompression reduced the stiffness of the distal forearm from 229.4 N/mm to 198.6 N/mm, there were minimal changes in the distribution of force in the radiocarpal and ulnocarpal fossa, suggesting no unloading of the lunate. The currently presumed benefit of core decompression is a response by the local vascular environment to trauma precipitating improved vascularity of the lunate. Although similar mechanisms for other procedures have been suggested by several investigators, evidence supporting this hypothesis is lacking. We do not use metaphyseal core decompression in our Kienböck disease treatment algorithm.

Intra-articular procedures requiring drilling of the lunate pose some challenges. In the surgical approach of the normal wrist, the lunate demonstrates minimal exposed dorsal surface with the wrist in neutral position. In the setting of Kienböck disease, with any degree of lunate collapse, the lunate often demonstrates even less exposed surface. Drilling for the purposes of decompression or creating a cortical window large enough to accommodate a vascularized bone flap (or vascular pedicle), requires wrist flexion and some resection of the cartilaginous surface of the proximal lunate. Making this window large enough to ensure that the bone flap maintains a robust connection to the vascular pedicle can require even greater resection of cartilage from the diseased lunate. We have found this intervention to be concerning, particularly in stage 3 Kienböck disease, where the structural integrity of the lunate is already tenuous. As stated earlier, our preference in early cases of Kienböck disease without collapse is to pursue lunate unloading. In cases demonstrating lunate collapse we feel that the unloading procedures are inadequate, and procedures requiring drilling or creating a cavity in the core of the collapsing lunate risk accelerating collapse. For this reason, although several procedures to revascularize the lunate have been described,[38,39,51–54] lunate decompression and vascularized bone/vessel insertion into the diseased lunate do not have any role in our algorithm.

More recently, medial femoral trochlea (MFT) osteochondral flap reconstruction of the proximal lunate provides a surgical option to revascularize the lunate and restore the proximal cartilaginous surface.[40,55] The initial reported series of MFT flaps used for Kienböck disease included 16 patients. Mean patient age was 35 and Lichtman staging was 2 in 7 patients, 3A in 8 patients, and 3B in 1 patient. Follow-up data included a minimum of 12 months after surgery. Computed tomography images obtained in patients confirmed healing in 15 of 16 patients, the Stahl indices remained unchanged, Lichtman staging remained unchanged in 10 patients, improved in 4 patients, and worsened in 2 patients (from 3A to 3B). Range of motion remained unchanged from preoperative measurements, whereas grip strength improved to 85% of the contralateral side. All but 1 patient demonstrated improvement in pain, with 12 having complete resolution of pain. More recently, Pet and colleagues[56] described the patient-reported outcomes after osteochondral reconstruction of the lunate. The mean DASH score was 10.8, and the mean Patient-Rated Wrist Evaluation score was 18.1. Outcomes reported reflected good postoperative patient health and function as well as low pain. The similarity of the MFT convex surface in the lunate fossa has also been examined demonstrating good congruity in radiographic and cadaveric studies.[57,58]

To date, our team has performed 46 cases of MFT reconstruction for Kienböck disease. The cases are primarily Lichtman stage 3A and 3B and we use this technique on Bain stage 1 and 2B Kienböck disease. If a patient demonstrates substantial collapse of the lunate, and the lunate fossa and proximal capitate are free of arthritis, we favor resection and replacement of the proximal capitate with the MFT convex osteochondral flap. As this flap provides only the proximal convex cartilage of the lunate, the concave distal lunate must be preserved. Fortunately, the progression of osteonecrosis of the lunate occurs from proximal to distal, permitting the use of this technique in patients with carpal collapse who have not progressed to midcarpal arthritis or degeneration of the lunate fossa. After resection of the collapsed proximal lunate, we are always able to encounter good-quality bone in the dorsal or volar horns of the distal native lunate permitting reconstruction.

Advanced Kienböck disease collapse is often accompanied by a coronal fracture into the acetabulum of the lunate (Bain 2B). As the fracture displaces, the volar and dorsal horns displace away from the coronal midline and progressively migrate distally. The dorsal fragment flexes, while the volar fragment extends. This phenomenon contributes to the widened dimensions measured as a decrease in the Stahl index. This disruption does not create a prominent surface facing the capitate,

and indeed, the 2 concave displaced surfaces support the convex capitate in a hammocklike fashion. Consequently, eburnation of the proximal capitate is rarely encountered. Because of this preservation of the capitate and lunate fossa, we include these collapsed and coronal fractured lunates among the cases of advanced Kienböck disease that may be capably reconstructed with MFT flap. After resection of the proximal lunate, reconstruction is performed by first reducing and fixing the midcarpal articulation, followed by insertion of the MFT to recapitulate the proximal lunate. This technique has been described in detail elsewhere.[59]

The MFT procedure provides the logical benefit of replacing the compromised lunate with structurally normal autograft and addressing the vascular etiology with a robust vascular pedicle. The analogous shape of the structures provides satisfying recreation of the lunate morphology both clinically and radiographically.[58] It also provides the opportunity to maintain the wrist's 2-joint articulation in young patients exhibiting advanced disease that would conventionally be treated with PRC.

We have narrowed our indications for MFT reconstruction to include those with stage 3A and 3B Kienböck disease who are skeletally mature, younger than age 40, and demonstrate a body mass index (BMI) less than 35. We have never performed this on skeletally immature patients to avoid risking femoral physis compromise. We have restricted our criteria to those younger than age 40 to avoid patients with any preexisting cartilaginous or meniscal knee pathology that predisposes the patient to donor site morbidity. Last, we have identified patients with a BMI greater than 34 as being at risk for demonstrating poorer scores on lower extremity patient-reported outcomes measures after MFT harvest, and therefore restrict our use of this technique to patients with a BMI less than 35.[56]

Salvage Procedures

In the category of salvage procedures, we would include all procedures eliminating 1 or both articulations of the wrist: PRC, partial wrist fusions, or total wrist fusion. Given the young age distribution of this disease process we would consider these options only in cases of severe arthritis and/or prior surgical failures.

Although the Lichtman and Bain staging system includes stage 4 as pancarpal arthritis, this is extremely rare in patients with Kienböck disease who are younger than 50. The capitate is often preserved because of the configuration of the lunate fragments described previously. Cases with substantial lunate collapse will also often demonstrate complete or partial preservation of lunate fossa cartilage. This may be due to the tendency of the lunate to collapse internally and maintain the continuity of the proximal convex cartilage shell. In these cases, the surgeon will encounter a lunate on exploration that seems less damaged than the radiographs indicate. The severe collapse may be appreciated only when manual pressure is applied to the proximal lunate surface and the lack of integrity becomes evident. Thus, total wrist fusion would only be considered in the elderly population with longstanding Kienböck disease that has deteriorated to pancarpal arthritis over decades of disease.

Partial wrist fusions reported for use in advanced Kienböck disease are aimed at offloading the lunate and transferring load across the radioscaphoid articulation.[41] Several intercarpal fusions have been described, including scapho-trapezial-trapezoid (STT), scaphocapitate (SC), and capitohamate fusions. These procedures may be done with or without lunate excision. While decreasing stress on the lunate, limited wrist arthrodesis has been shown to increase radioscaphoid forces significantly,[41] increasing the risk of arthritic progression in patients with SC or STT fusion. Although offloading procedures are generally accepted as the preferred procedure for early disease,[15] several studies have examined the results of intercarpal fusions in 3 A/B disease, with comparable results to other techniques. However, although reasonable short-term results have been demonstrated, the investigators acknowledge that the long-term effect on the radioscaphoid joint remained to be determined.[60–64] Indeed, Luegmair and Saffar[62] demonstrated secondary radioscaphoid arthritis in 50% of patients. These procedures seem to provide no advantage over a PRC, while carrying the risk of nonunion at the intercarpal fusion sites.

Our team uses the PRC as the salvage procedure in patients with lunate collapse who are older than 40 years or have a BMI greater than 35. We have also used PRC in 1 of our cohort of patients with MFT who failed to achieve adequate pain relief. Both Croog and Stern[65] and Lumsden and colleagues[66] have demonstrated comparable outcomes to other techniques in patients with Kienböck disease, demonstrating a postoperative average flexion-extension arc of 78% of the contralateral wrist with 87% maximal grip. Knowing the limitations in younger, more active patients questions the long-term viability of PRC for the management of Kienböck disease at younger ages.[67]

Alternative Procedures

In this category, we include synthetic lunate implant arthroplasty,[68–71] wrist denervation,[72–74] and arthroscopic synovectomy or drilling.[75,76] Of these, we have experience only with wrist denervation. This is typically done in the older population with advanced Kienböck disease, when the conventional treatment being considered is a salvage operation. Wrist denervation provides a low-morbidity alternative, where the surgeon may resect the anterior and posterior interosseous nerve via the same dorsal incision proximal to the distal radioulnar joint. In our experience, this routinely provides disappointing results with incomplete or no pain relief. Surgeons performing more complete wrist denervation may find more satisfying outcomes.

Lunate implant arthroplasty has the appeal of simplicity. However, given the typical presentation of Kienböck disease in a younger, active patient population, the inability to achieve any ligamentous stability of the implant has dissuaded us from using this modality.

Arthroscopic treatment of Kienböck disease is not included in our treatment algorithm. Arthroscopic evaluation for staging and planning purposes is commonly reported in the literature,[75,76] and some studies suggest varied interventions, such as synovectomy and arthrolysis, may provide benefit.[77,78]

A TREATMENT ALGORITHM FOR KIENBÖCK DISEASE

The common staging systems associated with Kienböck disease have been described in detail in this text elsewhere. The Lichtman classification combines radiographic parameters of perfusion, collapse, rotary instability, and arthritic changes into its rubric.[68] Bain and Begg's[79] articular-based classification describes the number of surfaces of the midcarpal and radiocarpal articulations that are damaged at the time of treatment. Lichtman classification remains the most commonly used by surgeons to determine treatment options, in conjunction with ulnar negative variance.[15] Our algorithm uses both of these in conjunction with the Bain classification.

A summary of our treatment algorithm is provided in **Box 1**. There are decision-making factors not listed on the figure that play a major role in decision making in each case. These include the patient's occupational and avocational demands, financial and time constraints, and social stressors. However, the general treatment pathways can be summarized as guidelines.

Box 1
Summary of treatment algorithm for Kienböck disease

Patients without collapse (or with minimal collapse of the lunate):

- <17 years of age
  - 12 weeks of cast immobilization
    - If failed trail of casting:
      - RSO (if ulnar negative)
      - CSO (if ulnar neutral or positive)
- >17 years of age
  - 12 weeks of cast immobilization (if they wish to trial nonsurgical management)
    - If interested in moving directly to surgical management or after failed trail of casting:
      - RSO (if ulnar negative)
      - CSO (if ulnar neutral or positive)

Patients with lunate collapse and no arthritis of the lunate fossa or capitate:

- Without coronal plane fracture into the lunate acetabulum
  - Age ≤40, BMI <35
    - Unloading RSO (if ulnar negative) or CSO (if ulnar neutral or positive)
    - MFT
  - Age >40 or BMI >34
    - Unloading RSO (if ulnar negative) or CSO (if ulnar neutral or positive)
    - PRC

With coronal plane fracture into the lunate acetabulum

- Age ≤40, BMI <35
  - MFT
- Age >40 or BMI >34
  - PRC

Patients >50 years of age with pancarpal arthritis

- Total wrist fusion

Abbreviations: BMI, body mass index; CSO, capitate shortening osteotomy; MFT, medial femoral trochlea; PRC, proximal row carpectomy; RSO, radial shortening osteotomy.

DISCLOSURE

The authors have nothing to disclose, such as no conflicts of interest, commercial associations, or intent of financial gain regarding this research.

REFERENCES

1. Bain GI, MacLean SB, Yeo CJ, et al. The etiology and pathogenesis of Kienbock disease. J Wrist Surg 2016;5(4):248–54.
2. Gelberman RH, Bauman TD, Menon J, et al. The vascularity of the lunate bone and Kienbock's disease. J Hand Surg Am 1980;5(3):272–8.
3. Panagis JS, Gelberman RH, Taleisnik J, et al. The arterial anatomy of the human carpus. Part II: The intraosseous vascularity. J Hand Surg Am 1983;8(4):375–82.
4. Lee ML. The intraosseus arterial pattern of the carpal lunate bone and its relation to avascular necrosis. Acta Orthop Scand 1963;33:43–55.
5. Schiltenwolf M, Martini AK, Mau HC, et al. Further investigations of the intraosseous pressure characteristics in necrotic lunates (Kienbock's disease). J Hand Surg Am 1996;21(5):754–8.
6. Jensen CH. Intraosseous pressure in Kienbock's disease. J Hand Surg Am 1993;18(2):355–9.
7. Hulten O. Über anatomische Variationen der Handgelenkknochen: Ein Beitrag zur Kenntnis der Genese zewi verschiedener Mondbeinver- anderungen. Act Radiol 1928;9:155–68.
8. Gelberman RH, Salamon PB, Jurist JM, et al. Ulnar variance in Kienbock's disease. J Bone Joint Surg Am 1975;57(5):674–6.
9. Bonzar M, Firrell JC, Hainer M, et al. Kienbock disease and negative ulnar variance. J Bone Joint Surg Am 1998;80(8):1154–7.
10. Afshar A, Aminzadeh-Gohari A, Yekta Z. The association of Kienbock's disease and ulnar variance in the Iranian population. J Hand Surg Eur Vol 2013;38(5):496–9.
11. Kristensen SS, Thomassen E, Christensen F. Ulnar variance in Kienbock's disease. J Hand Surg Br 1986;11(2):258–60.
12. Mirabello SC, Rosenthal DI, Smith RJ. Correlation of clinical and radiographic findings in Kienbock's disease. J Hand Surg Am 1987;12(6):1049–54.
13. Tsuge S, Nakamura R. Anatomical risk factors for Kienbock's disease. J Hand Surg Br 1993;18(1):70–5.
14. Stahl S, Stahl AS, Meisner C, et al. A systematic review of the etiopathogenesis of Kienbock's disease and a critical appraisal of its recognition as an occupational disease related to hand-arm vibration. BMC Musculoskelet Disord 2012;13:225.
15. Danoff JR, Cuellar DO, O J, et al. The management of Kienbock disease: a survey of the ASSH membership. J Wrist Surg 2015;4(1):43–8.
16. Lichtman DM, Lesley NE, Simmons SP. The classification and treatment of Kienbock's disease: the state of the art and a look at the future. J Hand Surg Eur Vol 2010;35(7):549–54.
17. Irisarri C, Kalb K, Ribak S. Infantile and juvenile lunatomalacia. J Hand Surg Eur Vol 2010;35(7):544–8.

18. Greene WB. Kienbock disease in a child who has cerebral palsy. a case report. J Bone Joint Surg Am 1996;78(10):1568–73.

19. Rasmussen F, Schantz K. Lunatomalacia in a child. Acta Orthop Scand 1987;58(1):82–4.

20. Kristensen SS, Thomassen E, Christensen F. Kienbock's disease–late results by non-surgical treatment. a follow-up study. J Hand Surg Br 1986; 11(3):422–5.

21. Taniguchi Y, Yoshida M, Iwasaki H, et al. Kienbock's disease in elderly patients. J Hand Surg Am 2003; 28(5):779–83.

22. Geutjens GG. Kienbock's disease in an elderly patient. J Hand Surg Am 1995;20(1):42–3.

23. Mikkelsen SS, Gelineck J. Poor function after nonoperative treatment of Kienbock's disease. Acta Orthop Scand 1987;58(3):241–3.

24. Viljakka T, Tallroth K, Vastamaki M. Long-term natural outcome (7-26 years) of Lichtman stage III Kienbock's lunatomalacia. Scand J Surg 2016;105(2): 125–32.

25. Werner FW, Murphy DJ, Palmer AK. Pressures in the distal radioulnar joint: effect of surgical procedures used for Kienbock's disease. J Orthop Res 1989; 7(3):445–50.

26. Trumble T, Glisson RR, Seaber AV, et al. A biomechanical comparison of the methods for treating Kienbock's disease. J Hand Surg Am 1986;11(1):88–93.

27. Salmon J, Stanley JK, Trail IA. Kienbock's disease: conservative management versus radial shortening. J Bone Joint Surg Br 2000;82(6):820–3.

28. Almquist EE, Burns JF Jr. Radial shortening for the treatment of Kienbock's disease–a 5- to 10-year follow-up. J Hand Surg Am 1982;7(4):348–52.

29. Weiss AP, Weiland AJ, Moore JR, et al. Radial shortening for Kienbock disease. J Bone Joint Surg Am 1991;73(3):384–91.

30. Rock MG, Roth JH, Martin L. Radial shortening osteotomy for treatment of Kienbock's disease. J Hand Surg Am 1991;16(3):454–60.

31. Rodrigues-Pinto R, Freitas D, Costa LD, et al. Clinical and radiological results following radial osteotomy in patients with Kienbock's disease: four- to 18-year follow-up. J Bone Joint Surg Br 2012;94(2):222–6.

32. Koh S, Nakamura R, Horii E, et al. Surgical outcome of radial osteotomy for Kienbock's disease-minimum 10 years of follow-up. J Hand Surg Am 2003;28(6): 910–6.

33. Raven EE, Haverkamp D, Marti RK. Outcome of Kienbock's disease 22 years after distal radius shortening osteotomy. Clin Orthop Relat Res 2007; 460:137–41.

34. Watanabe T, Takahara M, Tsuchida H, et al. Long-term follow-up of radial shortening osteotomy for Kienbock disease. J Bone Joint Surg Am 2008; 90(8):1705–11.

35. Matsui Y, Funakoshi T, Motomiya M, et al. Radial shortening osteotomy for Kienbock disease: minimum 10-year follow-up. J Hand Surg Am 2014; 39(4):679–85.

36. Benoliel R, Eliav E, Iadarola MJ. Neuropeptide Y in trigeminal ganglion following chronic constriction injury of the rat infraorbital nerve: is there correlation to somatosensory parameters? Pain 2001;91(1–2): 111–21.

37. van Leeuwen WF, Pong TM, Gottlieb RW, et al. Radial shortening osteotomy for symptomatic Kienbock's disease: complications and long-term patient-reported outcome. J Wrist Surg 2021;10(1):17–22.

38. Bochud RC, Buchler U. Kienbock's disease, early stage 3–height reconstruction and core revascularization of the lunate. J Hand Surg Br 1994;19(4): 466–78.

39. Ho Shin Y, Yoon JO, Ryu JJ, et al. Pronator quadratus pedicled bone graft in the treatment of Kienbock disease: follow-up 2 to 12 years. J Hand Surg Eur Vol 2020;45(4):396–402.

40. Higgins JP, Burger HK. The use of osteochondral flaps in the treatment of carpal disorders. J Hand Surg Eur Vol 2018;43(1):48–56.

41. Horii E, Garcia-Elias M, Bishop AT, et al. Effect on force transmission across the carpus in procedures used to treat Kienbock's disease. J Hand Surg Am 1990;15(3):393–400.

42. Kataoka T, Moritomo H, Omokawa S, et al. Decompression effect of partial capitate shortening for Kienbock's disease: a biomechanical study. Hand Surg 2012;17(3):299–305.

43. Werber KD, Schmelz R, Peimer CA, et al. Biomechanical effect of isolated capitate shortening in Kienbock's disease: an anatomical study. J Hand Surg Eur Vol 2013;38(5):500–7.

44. Almquist EE. Capitate shortening in the treatment of Kienbock's disease. Hand Clin 1993;9(3):505–12.

45. Afshar A, Mehdizadeh M, Khalkhali H. Short-term clinical outcomes of radial shortening osteotomy and capitates shortening osteotomy in Kienbock disease. Arch Bone Jt Surg 2015;3(3):173–8.

46. Rabarin F, Saint Cast Y, Cesari B, et al. [Capitate osteotomy in Kienbock's disease in twelve cases. Clinical and radiological results at five years follow-up]. Chir Main 2010;29(2):67–71. L'osteotomie du capitatum dans la maladie de Kienbock. Resultats cliniques et radiologiques a cinq ans de recul moyen. A propos de 12 cas.

47. Afshar A. Lunate revascularization after capitate shortening osteotomy in Kienbock's disease. J Hand Surg Am 2010;35(12):1943–6.

48. Atiyya AN, Nabil A, El Lattif AIA, et al. Partial capitate with/without hamate osteotomy in the treatment of Kienbock's disease: influence of the stage of the disease on the midterm outcome. J Wrist Surg 2020; 9(3):249–55.

49. Illarramendi AA, Schulz C, De Carli P. The surgical treatment of Kienbock's disease by radius and ulna metaphyseal core decompression. J Hand Surg Am 2001;26(2):252–60.

50. Sherman GM, Spath C, Harley BJ, et al. Core decompression of the distal radius for the treatment of Kienbock's disease: a biomechanical study. J Hand Surg Am 2008;33(9):1478–81.

51. Moran SL, Cooney WP, Berger RA, et al. The use of the 4 + 5 extensor compartmental vascularized bone graft for the treatment of Kienbock's disease. J Hand Surg Am 2005;30(1):50–8.

52. Sheetz KK, Bishop AT, Berger RA. The arterial blood supply of the distal radius and ulna and its potential use in vascularized pedicled bone grafts. J Hand Surg Am 1995;20(6):902–14.

53. Mathoulin C, Wahegaonkar AL. Revascularization of the lunate by a volar vascularized bone graft and an osteotomy of the radius in treatment of the Kienbock's disease. Microsurgery 2009;29(5):373–8.

54. Hori Y, Tamai S, Okuda H, et al. Blood vessel transplantation to bone. J Hand Surg Am 1979;4(1):23–33.

55. Higgins JP, Burger HK. Medial femoral trochlea osteochondral flap: applications for scaphoid and lunate reconstruction. Clin Plast Surg 2020;47(4):491–9.

56. Pet MA, Assi PE, Giladi AM, et al. Preliminary clinical, radiographic, and patient-reported outcomes of the medial femoral trochlea osteochondral free flap for lunate reconstruction in advanced Kienbock disease. J Hand Surg Am 2020;45(8):774 e1–8.

57. Hugon S, Koninckx A, Barbier O. Vascularized osteochondral graft from the medial femoral trochlea: anatomical study and clinical perspectives. Surg Radiol Anat 2010;32(9):817–25.

58. Van Handel AC, Lynch LM, Daruwalla JH, et al. Medial femoral trochlea flap reconstruction versus proximal row carpectomy for Kienbock's disease: a morphometric comparison. J Hand Surg Eur Vol 2021;46(10):1042–8.

59. Gillis JA, Higgins JP. Coronal fracture of the lunate in advanced Kienbock disease: reestablishing midcarpal congruency to enable osteochondral reconstruction: a case report. JBJS Case Connect 2018;8(2):e37.

60. Sauerbier M, Kluge S, Bickert B, et al. Subjective and objective outcomes after total wrist arthrodesis in patients with radiocarpal arthrosis or Kienbock's disease. Chir Main 2000;19(4):223–31.

61. Meier R, van Griensven M, Krimmer H. Scaphotrapeziotrapezoid (STT)-arthrodesis in Kienbock's disease. J Hand Surg Br 2004;29(6):580–4.

62. Luegmair M, Saffar P. Scaphocapitate arthrodesis for treatment of late stage Kienbock disease. J Hand Surg Eur Vol 2014;39(4):416–22.

63. Sennwald GR, Ufenast H. Scaphocapitate arthrodesis for the treatment of Kienbock's disease. J Hand Surg Am 1995;20(3):506–10.

64. Iorio ML, Kennedy CD, Huang JI. Limited intercarpal fusion as a salvage procedure for advanced Kienbock disease. Hand (N Y) 2015;10(3):472–6.

65. Croog AS, Stern PJ. Proximal row carpectomy for advanced Kienbock's disease: average 10-year follow-up. J Hand Surg Am 2008;33(7):1122–30.

66. Lumsden BC, Stone A, Engber WD. Treatment of advanced-stage Kienbock's disease with proximal row carpectomy: an average 15-year follow-up. J Hand Surg Am 2008;33(4):493–502.

67. Chim H, Moran SL. Long-term outcomes of proximal row carpectomy: a systematic review of the literature. J Wrist Surg 2012;1(2):141–8.

68. Alexander AH, Turner MA, Alexander CE, et al. Lunate silicone replacement arthroplasty in Kienbock's disease: a long-term follow-up. J Hand Surg Am 1990;15(3):401–7.

69. Bellemere P, Maes-Clavier C, Loubersac T, et al. Pyrocarbon interposition wrist arthroplasty in the treatment of failed wrist procedures. J Wrist Surg 2012;1(1):31–8.

70. Henry M. Outcomes assessment of lunate replacement arthroplasty with intrinsic carpal ligament reconstruction in Kienbock's disease. Hand (N Y) 2014;9(3):364–9.

71. Ma ZJ, Liu ZF, Shi QS, et al. Varisized 3D-printed lunate for Kienbock's disease in different stages: preliminary results. Orthop Surg 2020;12(3):792–801.

72. Fuchsberger T, Boesch CE, Tonagel F, et al. Patient-rated long-term results after complete denervation of the wrist. J Plast Reconstr Aesthet Surg 2018;71(1):57–61.

73. Schweizer A, von Kanel O, Kammer E, et al. Long-term follow-up evaluation of denervation of the wrist. J Hand Surg Am 2006;31(4):559–64.

74. Buck-Gramcko D. Wrist denervation procedures in the treatment of Kienbock's disease. Hand Clin 1993;9(3):517–20.

75. MacLean SBM, Bain GI. Long-term outcome of surgical treatment for Kienbock disease using an articular-based classification. J Hand Surg Am 2021;46(5):386–95.

76. Bain GI, MacLean SB, Tse WL, et al. Kienbock disease and arthroscopy: assessment, classification, and treatment. J Wrist Surg 2016;5(4):255–60.

77. Ayik O, Demirel M, Turgut N, et al. Arthroscopic debridement and arthrolysis for the treatment of advanced Kienbock's disease: 18-month and 5-year postoperative results. J Wrist Surg 2021;10(4):280–5.

78. Menth-Chiari WA, Poehling GG, Wiesler ER, et al. Arthroscopic debridement for the treatment of Kienbock's disease. Arthroscopy 1999;15(1):12–9.

79. Bain GI, Begg M. Arthroscopic assessment and classification of Kienbock's disease. Tech Hand Up Extrem Surg 2006;10(1):8–13.

Osteotomies, Core Decompression, and Denervation for the Treatment of Kienböck Disease

Kashyap K. Tadisina, MD, Mitchell A. Pet, MD*

KEYWORDS

• Kienböck disease • Radial shortening osteotomy • Wrist denervation • Core decompression

KEY POINTS

- Osteotomies, core decompression, and denervation all have demonstrated favorable outcomes in treatment of Kienböck disease, although this has been demonstrated mostly in the context of small or moderately sized case series.
- Radial shortening osteotomy is the most commonly reported surgical treatment used in Lichtman stage I, II, and IIIA with negative ulnar variance.
- Nonsalvage techniques (joint leveling, decompression) may preserve range of motion compared with salvage techniques in later-stage disease.
- Denervation has fallen out of favor, although prior case series have shown positive outcomes in later-stage disease.

INTRODUCTION

In this article, we review the operative treatment techniques of core decompression, various osteotomies, and denervation for Kienböck disease (KD). These techniques have been reported in varying stages of disease, including more advanced stages (Lichtman IIIA, IIIB, IV), in which ideal treatment modalities are often debated. Given the rarity of this disease, there is a dearth of high-level comparative studies to direct treatment. We review current indications, techniques, outcomes, and comparative studies across these 3 treatment modalities.

CORE DECOMPRESSION
Radius Core Decompression

Illarramendi and colleagues[1] first performed radius and ulna metaphyseal core decompressions

(MCD) in 1976. The original idea was borne after Illarramendi observed the resolution of symptoms in a patient with KD who had suffered an incidental distal radius fracture. The theoretic underpinning of this technique is that by creating a local controlled injury, MCD may increase blood flow to the nearby carpus via the arterial anastomotic system supplying the radius and carpus. Further, curettage may decrease intraosseous congestion and facilitate venous outflow. These forces in combination are thought to slow disease progression. Follow-up biomechanical studies offered some support to this theory, as it was found that core decompression does not alter radiolunate fossa loading. Rather, it was concluded that increased carpal vascularity is a more likely mechanism explaining the observed improvement after MCD.[2]

Initial techniques involved curettage of both the distal radius and ulna, but over time the radius has been more often treated alone. Illarramendi and

Department of Plastic and Reconstructive Surgery, Washington University in St. Louis, 660 S. Euclid Avenue. St Louis, MO 63110, USA
* Corresponding author.
E-mail address: mpet@wustl.edu

Hand Clin 38 (2022) 425–433
https://doi.org/10.1016/j.hcl.2022.03.006

colleagues[1] described a relatively simple dorsal approach to the wrist, periosteal elevation, cortical window creation, curettage with subsequent impaction of the radius that yielded favorable results clinically and radiologically at 10-year follow-up in their patient cohort. Advantages to MCD were the lack of complications associated with joint leveling procedures, including nonunion, distal radioulnar joint incongruence, ulnocarpal impingement, disruption of wrist kinematics, or problematic hardware. They advocated for this technique in patients with early-stage KD (stage 0, I, II). In their original report, they stated that results in stage 3A disease were not as robust as earlier stages, and 3B was a contraindication.[1]

The original article of Illarramendi and colleagues[1] reported on 22 patients with stage I to IIIA KD, average follow-up of 10 years, with 16 of 22 patients being pain free, average range of motion (ROM) 77%, and grip strength 75% of contralateral. Four patients who also had preoperative MRIs showed postoperative improvement in lunate vascularity. A subsequent follow-up study[3] examined 48 patients with an average follow-up of 9 years. In this series, 71% of patients were pain free, ROM for flexion/extension was 56°/60° compared with 77°/78° of the contralateral side, and grip strength was 75%. No patients had additional procedures performed, although 5 patients had unsatisfactory results.[3]

Adoption of Illaramendi's technique has yielded reproducible favorable long-term results in other published reports. De Carli and colleagues[4] followed 15 patients with Lichtman stage IIIA treated with radial MCD. At an average follow-up of 13 years, 14 patients had good or excellent results based on the modified Mayo wrist score. Mean visual analog scale (VAS) pain scores decreased from 7 preoperatively to 1.2 at final follow-up. Average ROM was 77% and grip strength 80% of contralateral side. Only 1 patient had a salvage proximal row carpectomy (PRC) performed. On radiographic examination, only 2 wrists progressed in Lichtman staging. Further, preoperative to postoperative modified carpal height ratio was 1.38 to 1.34, with only 3 patients demonstrating further carpal shortening.[4]

Lunate Core Decompression

Using a similar concept as radius core decompression, lunate core decompression has been proposed as another way to promote lunate revascularization.[5] Venous outflow obstruction and intraosseous congestion are thought to contribute to avascular necrosis pathogenesis. With direct curettage of the lunate, intraosseous pressure is decreased directly within the affected bone, facilitating venous outflow, while still recruiting the posttraumatic revascularization benefits mentioned previously. Mehrpour and colleagues[5] described this technique in 20 patients with stage I through IIIB KD. The open approach was described through a dorsal 2-cm incision directly over the lunate. Once through the extensor retinaculum and wrist capsule, a 2.5-mm burr was used to decompress the lunate. The investigators reported that after 5-year follow-up, VAS pain scores decreased from 88 to 14, Disability of the Arm, Shoulder, and Hand (DASH) scores decreased from 84 to 14, L = lunate tenderness decreased from 90% of patients to 15%, and ROM increased in wrist flexion (30° to 45°), extension (18° to 72°), radial (8° to 18°), and ulnar deviation (14° to 30°). Radiographically, no patients had progression of Lichtman stage or carpal height loss. Two patients with later-stage disease (IIIA, IIIB) went on to radial shortening osteotomy (RSO). The investigators concluded this as a viable technique comparable to joint leveling osteotomies with good medium-term outcomes in earlier-stage disease (stages I to II).[5]

Bain and colleagues[6] proposed lunate core decompression using an arthroscopic approach. Using the through 3, 4, and 6R portals, a 2-mm drill is used to decompress the lunate. Bain and colleagues[6] described 1 patient with early disease who had complete resolution of pain and no evidence of radiographic progression of disease at 6-year follow-up. The second patient had evidence of lunate sclerosis and collapse at presentation. Although this patient had resolution of pain, radiographic progression of disease was seen at 3-year and 6-year follow-up imaging. Based on these findings, the investigators reported that this technique may be best suited for patients with early-stage disease, ulnar neutral or positive variance, and preserved carpal height.[6] The potential complication of lunate fracture was mentioned in this report, although neither Mehrpour and colleagues[5] or Bain and colleagues[6] reported any complications.

OSTEOTOMIES

Osteotomies in the treatment of KD refers to a number of techniques meant to alter the biomechanics of load transmission across the carpus and radioulnar platform. The goal of these procedures in general is to decrease load on the lunate, thereby slowing/stopping its collapse and potentially facilitating revascularization.

A variety of techniques have been reported, including RSO, ulnar lengthening, closing/lateral wedge osteotomy of the radius, and capitate shortening. The most important consideration for choosing the appropriate osteotomy is ulnar variance. In the situation of negative ulnar variance, lunate offloading can be accomplished by shortening the radius or lengthening the ulna. When variance is neutral or positive, capitate shortening and radial closing/lateral wedge osteotomies are instead considered.

Radial Shortening

First introduced in 1981 by Martin and colleagues,[7] RSO is one of the most commonly performed osteotomy procedures. A 2016 survey study of American Society for Surgery of the Hand (ASSH) members revealed that RSO was the preferred surgical technique for Lichtman stage I, II, and IIIa with negative ulnar variance.[8] Biomechanical studies have shown that 2 to 3 mm of alteration provides relief, with any more than 4 mm contributing to instability of the radio-scaphoid joint. These studies estimated a 45% decrease in force across the radiolunate joint with radial shortening of 4 mm, and a 70% decrease in lunate strain with either technique. More specifically, it was noted that 90% of this decreased strain came with the first 2 mm of change in length.[9,10] Both dorsal and volar approaches have been described with specialized plates for these procedures.[11] Osteotomies can be made along the shaft or more distally along the metaphysis.

Long-term outcomes have been documented in several small series. Raven and colleagues[12] examined 11 patients who had RSO with an average of 22 years of follow-up. ROM was impaired compared with the contralateral side, with 79% to 103% in flexion/extension, 78% to 82% ulnar-radial deviation, and 93% to 99% prono-supination. Grip strength was 90% of the contralateral side (33 kg in treated hand compared with 37 kg in the untreated hand). Average VAS pain score was 2.4 and average DASH score was 14. Radiographic progression was absent in 8 patients. In 3 others, progression was observed, and was in each instance noted within the first 10 years postoperatively. The investigators of this study wrote that these findings represent reliable long-term results of RSO for stage I-IIIA KD.[12]

van Leeuwen and colleagues[13] examined reoperation rates in 48 patients with stage II or IIIA disease who underwent RSO. At an average follow-up time of 13 years, the rate of unplanned reoperations was 33% for the RSO group. Thirteen percent of RSO patients underwent PRC because of failure of RSO. QuickDASH scores were between 6.1 and 14, and pain scores were between 0.2 and 3.0 after RSO.[13] These results were compared with a cohort that underwent RSO and direct revascularization, with results indicating that there may be a benefit with direct revascularization.

Viljakka and colleagues[14] examined radiologic and clinical outcomes of 16 patients with stage 2, 3A, 3B disease treated with RSO with an average of 25 years of follow-up. Mean VAS pain scores were 0.9 at rest and 3.0 with heavy exertion. Mean ROM compared with contralateral hand was 88%, grip 95%, and key pinch was 107%. Lichtman stage was stable in 56% of patients. The investigators concluded that RSO provided 10-year sustained improvement in 75% of cases.[14]

The systematic review of Wang and colleagues[15] found that in patients with stage IIIA, radial shortening resulted in 26 of 27 patients being either pain free or with only mild pain on a VAS scale, ROM 68% to 88% of contralateral, and grip strength 70% to 79% of contralateral. For patients with stage IIIB, RSO resulted in 82% to 85% of contralateral ROM and 63% to 82% of contralateral grip strength.[15]

Ulnar Lengthening

Ulnar osteotomy with lengthening has been described as an alternative to RSO for ulnar negative wrists with KD. However this technique has fallen out of favor because of increased complication rates compared with RSO, and it is not recommended.[16,17]

CAPITATE SHORTENING OSTEOTOMY

Capitate shortening osteotomy (CSO) is a technique that has been applied for stages I, II, and IIIA KD with ulnar positive or neutral variance. In biomechanical studies, shortening the capitate has been found to decrease load on the lunate, with redistribution to the scaphotrapezial and triquetral-hamate joints.[10] In this technique, a dorsal approach to the wrist is used to access the capitate. A 1-mm to 2-mm transverse osteotomy is performed at the junction of the middle and distal third to avoid injury to the radioscaphocapitate and ulnocapitate ligament insertions. Fixation is typically achieved with headless compression screw or staples.[18,19] Partial capitate shortening is a variant technique that has been described. In this procedure, the trapezoid and scaphoid articulations, as well as radial length of the capitate, are preserved, while the lunate loading portion of the capitate is shortened.[20]

CSO was first reported by Almquist[21] in 1993, who reported a lunate revascularization rate of 83% after CSO with capitohamate fusion. Afshar[22] reported a series of 9 patients with stage II or IIIA disease who underwent capitate shortening. In this patient cohort, at an average follow-up of 12 months, all patients had partial or complete revascularization of the lunate. All patients had healing of the capitate osteotomy site by 6 weeks, and revascularization was reported at the 4.7 months postoperative mark.[22] Another study by Gay and colleagues[23] reviewed results of CSO in 11 patients with stage I-IIIA KD and neutral ulnar variance. At average follow-up of more than 5 years, mean VAS pain score was 1.7 and there was no change in ROM. Of these cases, 2 outcomes were deemed unacceptable by the patient, and revision procedures were performed.[23]

Distal Radial/Lateral/Closing Wedge Osteotomy

Closing wedge radial osteotomies have been proposed for patients with stage I-IIIA KD with ulnar positive or ulnar neutral variance. Some investigators have even advocated for this procedure without regard for ulnar variance.[24] The technique has been described since 1983[25,26] and uses an osteotomy to reduce the angle of radial inclination, thereby shifting load away from the lunate. Reducing radial inclination results in a radial shift of the vector of loading on the lunate. All of the carpal bones shift radially, with the capitate shifting the most, decreasing the load on the lunate, and transferring capitate load onto the scaphoid. Further, this shifts load from the triangular fibrocartilage to the more radial and stiffer articular cartilage of the radiolunate facet. Biomechanical analyses have found the ideal osteotomy wedge angle to be 15°.[25,26]

Miura and Sugioka[25] performed one of the first long-term outcome studies of this technique. The investigators examined 26 patients with KD of all stages and ulnar variance (negative, neutral, and positive) who underwent closing wedge osteotomy of the radius. At an average follow-up of more than 4 years, all patients had decreased pain, increased ROM, and increased grip strength. Based on the scoring system of Nakamura and colleagues,[27] 73% of patients had good or excellent results and 96% of patients were content with their results. When comparing patients with good/excellent results and those with fair/poor results, factors associated with a worse outcome were a higher preoperative radiolunate angle (17.7 vs 5.2°) and advanced stages of disease (IIIB or IV).[25,27]

This same group examined long-term results with a focus on radiographic analysis in 13 patients with an average of 14 years follow-up.[28] Radiographic analysis yielded a sustained decrease in radial inclination and increase in lunate covering ratio (amount of lunate covered by the radius), confirming a radial shift of the carpus. The amount of decrease in radial inclination was correlated with joint contact area of the lunate. Further analysis demonstrated that increased preoperative radiolunate and radioscaphoid angles (flexion deformity) did not resolve postoperatively with this technique. All patients had sustained improvement in pain, in addition to increased grip strength and ROM. Radiographic Lichtman stage advanced in 8 (57%) patients, was unchanged in 4 (29%), and improved in 1 (7%).[28]

Shin and colleagues[29] examined the results of radial wedge osteotomy in patients with late-stage KD. In this series, 14 patients with stage IIIA disease and 11 patients with stage IIIB or IV disease had radial wedge osteotomy performed. At an average follow-up of more than 7 years, favorable outcomes were found in both groups. In stage IIIA patients, 11 (79%) of 14 had radiologic improvement of the lunate. In stage IIIB and IV patients, 9 (82%) of 11 had radiologic improvement. Wrist ROM, grip strength, and DASH score improved in all patients, with no statistical difference between stage IIIA and stage IIIB/IV patient cohorts. The investigators concluded that radial wedge osteotomy could be a useful alternative to salvage procedures in later-stage KD.[29]

Other Osteotomies

A few other osteotomy techniques or combination techniques have been described. The reader should be aware of these techniques, but they are not the focus of this article. The modified Graner procedure includes lunate excision with capitate lengthening osteotomy and sometimes intercarpal arthrodesis.[30,31] Radial, ulnar, and capitate osteotomies also have been described in combination with a variety of bone grafts and intercarpal arthrodeses. However, there is a dearth of robust long-term or comparative data regarding these techniques.[11]

DENERVATION

Although wrist denervation has been performed for many decades, it appears that this technique has fallen out of favor with American surgeons according to surveys of ASSH members performed in 2012 and 2015 in the treatment of KD.[8,32] Most modern descriptions of denervation typically include the anterior interosseous nerve (AIN) and posterior interosseous nerve (PIN) as targets (**Figs. 1** and **2**).

Wrist denervation in KD was first mentioned in 1977 by Buck-Gramcko,[33] in a report about wrist denervation for a variety of pathologies. In this report, 32 patients were treated with wrist denervation at 6 or more specific anatomic sites with a follow-up of 4 years. A total of 10 different nerves were listed as targets for denervation:

1. PIN
2. The articular branch to the first intermetacarpal space (branch of superficial radial nerve)
3. The articular branches of the radial antebrachial cutaneous nerve
4. The superficial branch of the radial nerve
5. Palmar cutaneous branch of the median nerve
6. AIN
7 & 8. Dorsal distal perforating branches of the ulnar nerve (x2)
9. Dorsal cutaneous branch of the ulnar nerve (DCU)
10. Posterior antebrachial cutaneous nerve

In this series, 75% of patients were improved and satisfied, and 66% had no pain or pain only with manual labor. In a follow-up report in 1993, Buck-Gramcko[34] reviewed his outcomes specifically for the treatment of KD. He outlined a set of 47 patients for whom PIN denervation was performed as an adjunct to radial shortening, ulnar lengthening, lunate excision, lunate replacement with prosthesis or tendon, transposition of pisiform bone, or scaphotrapeziotrapezoid fusion. In this cohort, 27% of patients had no pain and 49% only had pain with manual work. In terms of satisfaction, 55% were very satisfied, 33% much improved, and 12% unsatisfied. Although no systematic comparison was performed, these satisfaction rates were higher than published operative technique outcomes of that time without denervation, supporting its use as an adjunctive technique.[34]

Denervation as a stand-alone treatment modality was performed in 14 patients in Buck-Gramcko's cohort,[34] some of whom had advanced disease. Denervation technique in these patients consisted of dividing 5 to 10 of the specific nerves listed previously. However, specific patient-level data were not included in this report. At 6.5 years of average follow-up, 88% of patients had some satisfaction with results. Complete pain relief was achieved in 3 patients (21%), 6 had pain only with manual labor (42%), and 3 had pain with daily activities (21%). A total of 3 patients had no relief of pain (21%). Radiographic progression was seen in 50%, grip strength had some improvement, and ROM was unaffected. Based on the symptomatic relief and high satisfaction rates, the investigator advocated for the use of partial or complete denervation in advanced stages of disease, either as an adjunct or primary procedure.[34]

Around this time in 1986, Ekerot and colleagues[35] published a review of 13 patients with stage III or IV KD who underwent complete wrist denervation. The goal of this study was to examine the radiographic progression of disease after

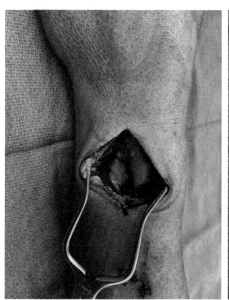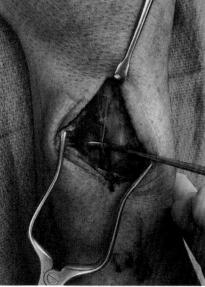

Fig. 1. After dorsal incision of the skin and extensor retinaculum, the terminal PIN is found in the base of the fourth extensor compartment.

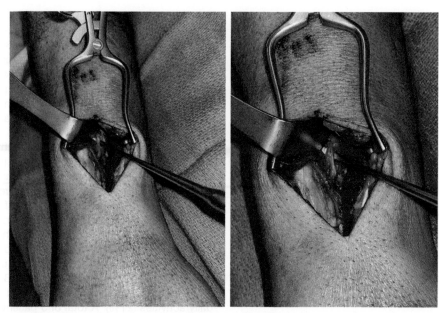

Fig. 2. After dividing the terminal PIN, a small window is created in the interosseous membrane. This allows access to and division of the terminal AIN.

denervation to evaluate if it had a detrimental effect on disease progression. Of the 13 patients, 7 had resolution of pain enough to go back to work after 4 years of follow-up, with the remaining 6 experiencing no relief. Further, radiographic follow-up led the investigators to conclude that denervation does not contribute to disease progression.[35]

Most recently in 2006, Schweizer and colleagues[36] performed a review of complete wrist denervation in their own series of 70 patients. The technique included denervation of 5 sites, including the AIN, PIN, DCU, the recurrent branch of the dorsoradial nerve to the index finger, and the recurrent dorsal cutaneous branches of the second and third webspaces. Of these 70 patients, 11 had denervation for KD. At an average follow-up of 9.6 years. 67% of all patients (including the KD cohort) reported improvement or resolution of pain.[36]

COMPARATIVE STUDIES

Literature comparing the preceding techniques that include rigorous study design and robust outcome measures are few in number, and represent an area of critical current interest.

A systematic review by Shin and colleagues[37] compared long-term outcomes of RSO and nonoperative treatment. In this review, it was found that RSO had improved outcomes with regard to pain and ROM, but was no better compared with conservative management with regard to radiographic disease progression. The

investigators noted the lack of high-quality evidence in their analysis, and recommended prospective studies to help surgeons accurately make informed management decisions.[37]

Kamrani and colleagues[38] performed a prospective study with 64 patients and compared arthroscopic lunate core decompression and synovectomy versus radial osteotomies (shortening in ulnar negative wrists and wedge osteotomy in ulnar positive) for patients with stage I-IIIB KD. At a mean follow-up of 3 years, QuickDASH, VAS pain scores, and ROM improved in all groups, whereas strength increased significantly only in the decompression group. There were no significant differences on postoperative functional analysis outside of passive wrist extension (which was more favorable in the decompression group). The investigators concluded that radial osteotomies and lunate core decompression had comparable results at intermediate-term follow-up.[38]

Iwasaki and colleagues[39] performed a comparative study of radial shortening and wedge osteotomies in 20 patients with late-stage (IIIB and IV) disease. After 2.4 years of follow-up, both procedures yielded good or excellent outcomes. The wedge osteotomy group had 2 patients with radiographic progression compared with zero patients in the shortening group. The investigators concluded comparable results between techniques at short-term follow-up.[39]

Recent systematic reviews have separated patient cohorts into early-stage (I-IIIA) and late-stage (IIIB and IV) disease in an attempt to analyze existing literature.[15,40] The conclusions from these studies with respect to decompression and osteotomy were unable to identify a clearly superior technique in early-stage KD, with all interventions showing improvement in pain and ROM and insufficient data for further analysis.[40] In more advanced disease, joint leveling and radial wedge osteotomies were found to preserve greater ROM compared with salvage techniques (arthrodesis, PRC, arthroplasty).[15]

SUMMARY

The studies summarized in this article represent the accumulated evidence that underpins the use of decompression, osteotomy, and denervation for the treatment of KD. Although much has been learned, the evidence consists mostly of case series and uncontrolled comparative studies, which use variable language, indications, and measures of outcome. Although tightly controlled comparative studies are certainly needed, the relative rarity of KD makes this quite difficult to accomplish in isolation. In the future, it is our hope that pertinent questions in this field will be addressed as a national or international collaborative effort. It is with these limitations of current evidence in mind that we offer how we have incorporated decompression, osteotomy, and denervation into our practice.

Although decompression has some appeal as an extra-articular, relatively simple intervention for the treatment of KD, we do not routinely perform this as a stand-alone procedure. We find that the current theoretic underpinnings of this procedure (increased local perfusion and intraosseous decongestion) are not necessarily intuitive, and are likely incompletely understood. Furthermore, given our positive experience with lunate revascularization using 4, 5 extracompartmental artery pedicled vascularized bone flap (in stage II or early IIIA disease, especially with ulnar neutral or positive variance),[41] we have been hesitant to interrupt the subchondral and metaphyseal bone that is intrinsic to or near the potential flap donor site. That said, it could be interpreted that any bone graft/flap harvest from the distal radius could constitute a sort of MCD, and it remains possible that some of the favorable outcomes we have seen after pedicled bone flap reconstruction of the lunate could be attributable to the inherent MCD, at least in part.

With regard to osteotomy, we have generally made use only of metaphyseal RSO. We have found this useful in some situations of stage I, II, and early IIIA KD with ulnar negative variance. This extra-articular procedure has a relatively low complication rate, is easy to perform, and is amenable to relatively rapid rehabilitation. In situations of ulnar neutral or positive variance with relatively preserved lunate integrity and carpal alignment, we have generally favored lunate revascularization as the primary bony procedure. As such, we have limited experience with radial wedge or CSO. In particular, we prefer to avoid manipulation of an intact capitate, recognizing that PRC may be useful for many patients with KD at some point. In our opinion, maintenance of a native and untouched capitate is desirable, as the outcomes of PRC after CSO (complicated or uncomplicated) are not known.

It is our interpretation of the preceding evidence that wrist denervation likely has a role as a stand-alone and/or adjunctive treatment for KD. We routinely perform AIN and PIN neurectomy through a single dorsal approach (see **Figs. 1** and **2**) when performing RSO, lunate revascularization, lunate reconstruction, and wrist salvage. In addition, we have offered this low-risk extra-articular procedure for patients with KD who are poorly suited or hesitant to undergo bony surgery. However, although we do use this technique in practice, it is undeniable that existing outcomes data cannot be considered conclusive in favor of efficacy.

Given our incomplete understanding regarding the etiology of KD and the efficacy of the treatments discussed, we have generally chosen to discuss the logic and evidence supporting available surgical options in detail with each patient. Just as the different treatment modalities may have unique appeal to different surgeons, we have found that patients often find resonance with some options and not others. Finally, the options discussed here must be considered in the context of the other methodologies discussed in this volume, as a large and flexible toolbox is advantageous in treating this perplexing disease.

CLINICS CARE POINTS

- Core decompression has shown favorable outcomes, and can be considered for early stage KD. However, the mechanism of action is poorly understood.

- Radial shortening osteotomy is primarily indicated for early stage KD with ulnar negative variance. Some series have suggested efficacy in advanced cases.

- Capitate shortening and radial wedge osteotomy are primarily used in cases of KD with ulnar neutral or positive variance.

• A wide variety of denervation procedures have been advocated for KD. These may be employed as standalone or adjunctive interventions.

REFERENCES

1. Illarramendi AA, Schulz C, De Carli P. The surgical treatment of Kienböck's disease by radius and ulna metaphyseal core decompression. J Hand Surg Am 2001;26(2):252–60.
2. Sherman GM, Spath C, Harley BJ, et al. Core decompression of the distal radius for the treatment of Kienböck's disease: a biomechanical study. J Hand Surg Am 2008;33(9):1478–81.
3. Illarramendi AA, De Carli P. Radius decompression for treatment of Kienböck disease. Tech Hand Up Extrem Surg 2003;7(3):110–3.
4. De Carli P, Zaidenberg EE, Alfie V, et al. Radius core decompression for Kienböck disease stage IIIA: outcomes at 13 years follow-up. J Hand Surg Am 2017;42(9):752.e1–6.
5. Mehrpour SR, Kamrani RS, Aghamirsalim MR, et al. Treatment of Kienböck disease by lunate core decompression. J Hand Surg Am 2011;36(10):1675–7.
6. Bain GI, Smith ML, Watts AC. Arthroscopic core decompression of the lunate in early stage Kienbock disease of the lunate. Tech Hand Up Extrem Surg 2011;15(1):66–9.
7. Martin R, Veldstra R, Vegter J. Shortening osteotomy of the radius in the treatment of Kienbock's disease. Orthopade 1981;10:54–8.
8. Danoff JR, Cuellar DO, O J, et al. The management of Kienböck disease: a survey of the ASSH membership. J Wrist Surg 2015;4(1):43–8 [Erratum appears in: J Wrist Surg. 2015 May;4(2):148].
9. Trumble T, Glisson RR, Seaber AV, et al. A biomechanical comparison of the methods for treating Kienböck's disease. J Hand Surg Am 1986;11(1):88–93.
10. Horii E, Garcia-Elias M, An KN, et al. Effect on force transmission across the carpus in procedures used to treat Kienböck's disease. J Hand Surg Am 1990;15:393–400.
11. Lee SK. Fractures of the carpal bones. In: Wolfe SW, Pederson WC, Kozin SH, editors. Green's operative hand surgery. Philadelphia, PA: Elsevier/Churchill Livingstone; 2016. p. 636–49.
12. Raven EE, Haverkamp D, Marti RK. Outcome of Kienböck's disease 22 years after distal radius shortening osteotomy. Clin Orthop Relat Res 2007;460:137–41.
13. van Leeuwen WF, Pong TM, Gottlieb RW, et al. Radial shortening osteotomy for symptomatic Kienböck's disease: complications and long-term patient-reported outcome. J Wrist Surg 2021;10(1):17–22.
14. Viljakka T, Tallroth K, Vastamäki M. Long-term outcome (20 to 33 years) of radial shortening osteotomy for Kienböck's lunatomalacia. J Hand Surg Eur Vol 2014;39(7):761–9.
15. Wang PQ, Matache BA, Grewal R, et al. Treatment of stages IIIA and IIIB in Kienbock's disease: a systematic review. J Wrist Surg 2020;9(6):535–48.
16. Cross D, Matullo KS. Kienböck disease. Orthop Clin North Am 2014;45(1):141–52.
17. Netto AP, Szabo RM. Radial-shortening and ulnar-lengthening operations for Kienböck's disease. In: Lichtman D, Bain G, editors. Kienböck's disease. Cham: Springer; 2016.
18. Hunter AR, Temperley D, Trail IA. Capitate shortening osteotomy and vascularized bone grafting for Kienböck's disease in ulnar positive or neutral wrists. J Hand Surg Eur Vol 2021;46(6):581–6.
19. Hegazy G, Seddik M, Massoud AH, et al. Capitate shortening osteotomy with or without vascularized bone grafting for the treatment of early stages of Kienböck's disease. Int Orthop 2021;45(10):2635–41.
20. Singer MS, Essawy OM, Farag HE. Early results of partial capitate shortening osteotomy in management of Kienböck disease. Curr Orthop Pract 2017;28:297–302.
21. Almquist EE. Capitate shortening in the treatment of Kienböck's disease. Hand Clin 1993;9(3):505–12.
22. Afshar A. Lunate revascularization after capitate shortening osteotomy in Kienböck's disease. J Hand Surg Am 2010;35(12):1943–6.
23. Gay AM, Parratte S, Glard Y, et al. Isolated capitate shortening osteotomy for the early stage of Kienböck disease with neutral ulnar variance. Plast Reconstr Surg 2009;124(2):560–6.
24. Rioux-Forker D, Shin AY. Osteonecrosis of the lunate: Kienböck disease. J Am Acad Orthop Surg 2020;28(14):570–84.
25. Miura H, Sugioka Y. Radial closing wedge osteotomy for Kienböck's disease. J Hand Surg Am 1996;21(6):1029–34.
26. Tsumura H, Himeno S, Morita H, Sasaki Y, et al. The optimum correcting angle of wedge osteotomy at the distal end of the radius for Kienbock's disease. J Jap Soc Surg Hand 1984;I:435–9.
27. Nakamura R, Imaeda T, Miura T. Radial shortening for Kienböck's disease: factors affecting the operative result. J Hand Surg Br 1990;15(1):40–5.
28. Wada A, Miura H, Kubota H, et al. Radial closing wedge osteotomy for Kienböck's disease: an over 10 year clinical and radiographic follow-up. J Hand Surg Br 2002;27(2):175–9.
29. Shin YH, Kim J, Gong HS, et al. Clinical outcome of lateral wedge osteotomy of the radius in advanced

stages of Kienböck's disease. Clin Orthop Surg 2017;9(3):355–62.

30. Li J, Pan Z, Zhao Y, et al. Capitate osteotomy and transposition for type III Kienböck's disease. J Hand Surg Eur Vol 2018;43(7):708–11.

31. Graner O, Lopes EI, Carvalho BC, et al. Arthrodesis of the carpal bones in the treatment of Kienböck's disease, painful ununited fractures of the navicular and lunate bones with avascular necrosis, and old fracture-dislocations of carpal bones. J Bone Joint Surg Am 1966;48(4):767–74.

32. Stahl S, Santos Stahl A, Rahmanian-Schwarz A, et al. An international opinion research survey of the etiology, diagnosis, therapy and outcome of Kienböck's disease (KD). Chir Main 2012;31(3):128–37.

33. Buck-Gramcko D. Denervation of the wrist joint. J Hand Surg Am 1977;2(1):54–61.

34. Buck-Gramcko D. Wrist denervation procedures in the treatment of Kienböck's disease. Hand Clin 1993;9(3):517–20.

35. Ekerot L, Jonsson K, Necking LE. Wrist denervation and compression of the lunate in Kienböck's disease. Scand J Plast Reconstr Surg 1986;20(2):225–7.

36. Schweizer A, von Känel O, Kammer E, et al. Long-term follow-up evaluation of denervation of the wrist. J Hand Surg Am 2006;31(4):559–64.

37. Shin YH, Kim JK, Han M, et al. Comparison of long-term outcomes of radial osteotomy and nonoperative treatment for Kienböck disease: a systematic review. J Bone Joint Surg Am 2018;100(14):1231–40.

38. Kamrani RS, Najafi E, Azizi H, et al. Outcomes of arthroscopic lunate core decompression versus radial osteotomy in treatment of Kienböck disease. J Hand Surg Am 2021;21:S0363–5023, 00449-4.

39. Iwasaki N, Minami A, Oizumi N, et al. Radial osteotomy for late-stage Kienböck's disease. Wedge osteotomy versus radial shortening. J Bone Joint Surg Br 2002;84(5):673–7.

40. Innes L, Strauch RJ. Systematic review of the treatment of Kienböck's disease in its early and late stages. J Hand Surg Am 2010;35(5):713–7, 717.e1-717.

41. Moran SL, Cooney WP, Berger RA, et al. The use of the 4 + 5 extensor compartmental vascularized bone graft for the treatment of Kienböck's disease. J Hand Surg Am 2005;30(1):50–8.

Vascularized Bone Flaps for the Treatment of Kienböck Disease

Matthew M. Florczynski, FRCSC, MD, MS[a], Kevin C. Chung, MD, MS[a,b],*

KEYWORDS

- Free osteochondral flap • Kienböck disease • Lunate revascularization • Pedicled bone flap

KEY POINTS

- The vascular anatomy of the carpus can be conceptualized as a communicating series of longitudinal supplying vessels and transverse arches in forming a redundant blood supply to the bone.
- Compared to nonvascularized grafts, the use of vascularized bone flaps to treat osteonecrosis results in more rapid regeneration of bone and improved cartilage quality when osteochondral flaps are used.
- Pedicled 4,5 extracompartmental artery and metacarpal base flaps are preferred treatments for lunate osteonecrosis with preserved articular cartilage.
- Free osseocartilaginous flaps are indicated when osteonecrosis has occurred and the proximal lunate articular surface has been compromised.

INTRODUCTION

Over a century after Robert Kienböck coined the term lunatomalacia to describe radiographic changes from lunate osteonecrosis, the disorder with his namesake remains one of the great dilemmas in hand surgery.[1] Kienböck disease is a rare condition with an estimated prevalence ranging from less than 0.01% to 0.27%.[2,3] Its etiology is likely multifactorial, resulting from the interplay of vascular, mechanical, metabolic, and genetic factors.[4–6] Although historically there was debate about the natural history of Kienböck disease, studies have demonstrated a predictable relationship between the passage of time and progression of disease.[7–9] Radiographic changes and fragmentation of the lunate can occur within 6 months of the onset of symptoms, and though

conventional treatments may improve symptoms, they do not alter the natural progression of disease.[10,11] Of the many surgical treatments available, only lunate revascularization has the potential to reverse the pathologic changes in Kienböck disease. With the advent of new techniques, indications for lunate revascularization are expanding and offer a promising solution for patients with previously unreconstructible lunate degeneration.

VASCULAR ANATOMY OF THE CARPUS

Osteonecrosis of the lunate has been linked to impaired vascularity in attempts to explain the pathophysiology of Kienböck disease. Early theories posited that a compression fracture results in disruption of the intraosseous blood supply

Disclosure: Dr Chung received funding from the National Institutes of Health and book royalties from Wolters Kluwer and Elsevier. Research reported in this publication was supported by the National Institute of Arthritis and Musculoskeletal and Skin Diseases of the National Institutes of Health under Award Number U01-AR073485. The content is solely the responsibility of the authors and does not necessarily represent the official views of the National Institutes of Health.

[a] Section of Plastic Surgery, Department of Surgery, University of Michigan Medical School, Ann Arbor, MI, USA; [b] Comprehensive Hand Center Michigan Medicine, 2130 Taubman Center, SPC 5340, 1500 E. Medical Center Drive, Ann Arbor, MI 48109-5340, USA
* Corresponding author. Comprehensive Hand Center Michigan Medicine, 2130 Taubman Center, SPC 5340, 1500 E. Medical Center Drive, Ann Arbor, MI 48109-5340.
E-mail address: kecchung@umich.edu

0749-0712/22/© 2022 Elsevier Inc. All rights reserved.

and subsequent osteonecrosis.[12,13] It was later postulated that lunate offloading procedures protect the lunate from fracture and osteonecrosis.[14] It is now clear that not all cases of Kienböck disease are precipitated by lunate fracture. Subsequent theories focused on natural variations in the arterial supply to the lunate and predisposition of particular vascular patterns to osteonecrosis.[15,16] Others suggested that increased intraosseous pressure impairs venous outflow and results in lunate osteonecrosis.[17,18] Although these hypotheses are reasonable, they have not been substantiated clinically.[4,19] Nevertheless, they have improved our understanding of the vascular anatomy of the lunate, which is central to the treatment of Kienböck disease.

Detailed knowledge of the vascular anatomy of the forearm and carpal bones is important for understanding lunate revascularization procedures. The radial, ulnar, and anterior interosseous artery (AIA), as well as lesser contributions from the deep palmar arch and recurrent branches of the ulnar artery, feed a series of dorsal and volar transverse arches that provide the extraosseous blood supply to the carpus.[15,20,21] A thorough analysis of the blood supply to the lunate was performed in a classic study by Gelberman and colleagues[15] Dorsally, 3 arches were found to contribute to the vascularity of the lunate. The dorsal radiocarpal arch was the most proximal and gave off nutrient vessels to the lunate and triquetrum. The dorsal intercarpal arch, traversing between the proximal and distal carpal rows, was the largest and most ubiquitous and supplied the distal carpal row, lunate, and triquetrum. The basal metacarpal arch was the most distal, smallest, and variably present. A similar pattern of volar arches was identified. The palmar radiocarpal and deep palmar arches were found to be present consistently, whereas the palmar intercarpal arch was only present in 53% of specimens and provided the smallest contribution. This system of longitudinal vessels communicating through transverse arches also supplies the distal radius, ulna, and metacarpal bones.[20,22] Taking advantage of this intricate structure, a variety of pedicled flaps can be designed to fit defects in the lunate.[23,24] The redundancy of this blood supply also facilitates safe anastomosis of free vascularized osteochondral flaps to recipient vessels.[21,25]

ROLE OF LUNATE REVASCULARIZATION IN THE TREATMENT OF KIENBÖCK DISEASE

Following the onset of osteonecrosis, a sequence of biologic events called "creeping substitution" is initiated, in which necrotic bone is resorbed and replaced by new bone.[26] This process is characterized by a relative predominance of osteoclast-mediated bone resorption compared with osteoblast-mediated bone formation.[4] As osteonecrosis progresses, the bone becomes vulnerable to subchondral fracture, precipitating irreversible degenerative changes. Nonvascularized bone grafts promote bone healing through this mechanism.[27] Contrastingly, vascularized bone flaps bypass the creeping substitution mechanism and are consolidated more rapidly with less resorption.[28,29]

Rationale for Vascularized Bone Flaps

The superiority of vascularized bone flaps over nonvascularized grafts has been demonstrated in animal models. Owing to similarities in the anatomy of the distal radius, canine models have been used to study osteonecrosis of the proximal pole of the scaphoid. Compared with nonvascularized grafts, reverse-flow vascularized pedicled flaps increased blood flow to the previously necrotic area and demonstrated higher levels of trabecular osteoblasts and osteoid on histologic analysis.[30,31] Hori and colleagues[32] demonstrated neovascularization and new bone formation after transplanting an isolated neurovascular bundle into the canine tibia. They subsequently described their successes with this technique in 9 cases of Kienböck disease; however, the purported salutary outcomes of vascular bundle implantation to the necrotic lunate have not been replicated.

The effects of free osseocartilaginous bone flaps on cartilage regeneration have also been studied. Articular cartilage is thought to rely primarily on synovial imbibition rather than intraosseous supply for blood flow. Higgins and colleagues[33] performed a study using pigs in which they implanted either nonvascularized or free vascularized osteochondral flaps into articular distal femur bone defects lined with methylmethacrylate cement to prevent communication between subchondral bone at the recipient site and the transplanted bone. After 6 months, the vascularized osteochondral flaps demonstrated superior cartilage surface quality and a greater percentage of viable chondrocytes. Although vascularized flaps formed new hyaline cartilage, the surface of nonvascularized grafts was composed of hyaline and fibrocartilage. Although treatments for Kienböck disease are generally meant to halt disease progression, vascularized bone flaps can potentially reverse changes caused by osteonecrosis and restore native functional anatomy.

Indications for Lunate Revascularization

With recent advances in revascularization techniques, salvage procedures should no longer be considered the only option for patients with advanced Kienböck disease. Vascularized pedicled bone flaps can be considered to replace necrotic subchondral bone any time the surrounding cartilage surface of the lunate is preserved. They can be used in conjunction with lunate unloading procedures to replace the existing bone loss and protect against future subchondral fractures due to radiocarpal contact. The indications for free vascularized osteochondral flaps are broader because they can be used to replace the degenerate proximal articular surface of the lunate in conjunction with an underlying bone defect. The use of pedicled and free vascularized bone flaps has been reported for Lichtman stages I through IIIC.[5] These techniques can also be used together with partial wrist fusions as an alternative to other salvage procedures.

EVALUATION OF OSTEONECROSIS OF THE LUNATE

As many patients with Kienböck disease are asymptomatic, the initial assessment must include a thorough clinical examination to rule out other causes of wrist symptoms. Patients typically present with unilateral progressive symptoms of insidious onset, characterized by dorsal, central wrist pain and swelling, and subtle decreases in wrist motion. Special attention should be paid to the duration of symptoms, as this has prognostic importance.[7–9] Standard wrist radiographs are the initial imaging modality of choice and the basis for the Lichtman classification.[34] Although radiographs are insensitive in early disease, lunate pathology may be detectable earlier than previously thought.[11] Osteonecrosis has a characteristic appearance with patchy densities and sclerosis, and making the diagnosis on radiographs may obviate the need for more costly advanced imaging.[35]

Role of Advanced Imaging Studies

Two advanced imaging modalities typically considered for preoperative evaluation of Kienböck disease are computed tomography (CT) and MRI. CT is useful in late disease for evaluating bone stock and subchondral fractures.[36] CT is also superior to other modalities for detecting specific lunate morphologies (ie, presence or absence of a medial hamate facet), which may have prognostic importance.[37] A recent study showed that the lunate width-to-height ratio measured on CT

was a better predictor of carpal collapse than indices commonly measured on x-rays, such as ulnar variance and carpal height.[38] Careful preoperative evaluation of bony detail can be helpful in planning the site of bone graft harvest and estimating the amount of graft needed.

MRI is superior to other imaging modalities for the detection of early osteonecrosis.[35,39] T1-weighted images show a characteristic decrease in signal density thought to correspond to physiologic changes associated with creeping substitution. However, small areas of osteonecrosis may still be difficult to detect and T2-weighted images are often unremarkable. More importantly, the relevance of the MRI finding of avascularity to bone healing potential is not clearly defined.[40] Given these limitations, we recommend intraoperative evaluation of the carpal anatomy before proceeding with revascularization.

Role of Arthroscopy

Studies have called into question the reliability of radiographic classifications of Kienböck disease.[41,42] Imaging modalities fare particularly poorly in the assessment of articular cartilage of the carpus. Wrist arthroscopy has become the new standard for the assessment of articular surfaces of the lunate and the wrist.[43] Bain and Begg[44] developed an arthroscopic classification of Kienböck disease to guide surgical management based on the number of functional and nonfunctional articular surfaces surrounding the lunate. Functional articular surfaces were defined as smooth and glistening in appearance, whereas nonfunctional surfaces had degenerative changes such as synovitis, fraying, or fracture. They proposed a treatment algorithm based on these findings, and subsequent combined classifications and treatment algorithms based on similar principles have been developed.[45,46] Although arthroscopic classifications have their own shortcomings, the integrity of the lunate cartilage is central to determining the appropriate lunate revascularization procedure. Furthermore, arthroscopy can be used to assist or substitute certain open procedures, such as lunate decompression, limited wrist fusions, or proximal row carpectomy.[43]

TREATMENT OF KIENBÖCK DISEASE WITH LUNATE REVASCULARIZATION

The treatment of Kienböck disease with lunate revascularization can be divided into 2 categories of procedures. Vascularized bone flaps made up of corticocancellous bone can be used to reconstruct necrotic defects in the lunate, as long as an intact cartilage shell has been preserved.[47] These flaps are mostly pedicled, afforded by the redundant vascular anatomy of the carpus. Advantages of pedicled vascularized bone flaps include potential for rapid revascularization that bypasses the normal creeping substitution mechanism, using only one surgical incision with minimal donor site morbidity, and relative technical ease without need for microsurgery or articular reconstruction. The second category of lunate revascularization procedures requires reconstruction of subchondral and articular defects in the lunate using free osseocartilaginous flaps.

Pedicled Distal Radius Flaps

Use of a pedicled vascularized bone flap can be considered any time there is lunate bone loss with a preserved cartilage shell. Numerous pedicled vascularized bone flaps have been described based on the local anatomy of the hand and wrist.[22,23,47,48] The radial artery and AIA are the main feeding vessels to the dorsal distal radius and give off 4 main branches (**Fig. 1**). Each of these arteries is numbered based on its adjacent extensor tendon compartments, with the intracompartmental supraretinacular arteries (ICSRAs) traveling superficial to the extensor retinaculum and the extracompartmental arteries (ECAs) traveling deep along the floor of their extensor compartments. Owing to their radial location, flaps based on the 1,2 and 2,3 ICSRAs are commonly used in reconstruction of the proximal pole of the scaphoid. They can also be used in Kienböck disease, particularly the 2,3 ICSRA for its longer excursion.[49] Lunate revascularization with a pedicled pisiform flap has also been studied but is mostly of historical interest because of poor long-term outcomes.[50]

The 4,5 ECA flap has become a workhorse pedicled flap in Kienböck disease. It is often used in conjunction with a radial shortening osteotomy as a lunate unloading procedure in patients with ulnar negative wrists. The fourth ECA originates from the posterior division of the AIA, runs along the radial side of the floor of the fourth extensor compartment, and connects with the dorsal radiocarpal and intercarpal arches. The fifth ECA, which is the largest of the dorsal vessels, originates from the posterior division of the AIA and forms multiple anastomoses distally, including the fourth ECA. Although either the fourth or fifth ECAs can be used as pedicles on their own, incorporating both vessels increases the excursion of the pedicle considerably.[23]

One surgical technique we have done in patients with ulnar negative wrists and preserved lunate

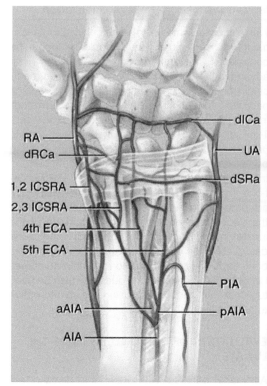

Fig. 1. Detailed anatomy of the dorsal distal radius demonstrating longitudinal feeding vessels (AIA, anterior interosseous artery; PIA, posterior interosseous artery; RA, radial artery; UA, ulnar artery) and communicating transverse arches (dICa, dorsal intercarpal arch; dRCa, dorsal radiocarpal arch; dSRa, dorsal supraretinacular arch). Four main vessel branches used for pedicled vascularized bone flaps are also shown (4th and 5th ECA, extracompartmental artery; 1,2 and 2,3 ICSRA, intracompartmental supraretinacular artery). aAIA and pAIA are anterior and posterior divisions of the anterior interosseous artery. (*From* Elhassan BT, Shin AY. Vascularized bone grafting for treatment of Kienböck disease. J Hand Surg Am. 2009;34(1):148; with permission)

articular cartilage is to use the 4,5 ECA flap in conjunction with a radial shortening osteotomy. Owing to the close proximity of the flap to the lunate, we do not typically inspect the lunate arthroscopically for this procedure. If arthroscopy is used, the 4,5 and ulnar midcarpal portals should be avoided because of the risk of injury to the fourth and fifth ECAs.[23] Instead, the 6U and 6R portals can be used as working portals, together with standard 3,4 and radial midcarpal viewing portals. Under a regional block with tourniquet control, we use a longitudinal midline incision made dorsally (**Fig. 2**A, B). Full-thickness skin flaps are elevated and a longitudinal or ligament-sparing arthrotomy is made over the carpus.[51] The lunate articular surface is inspected and the

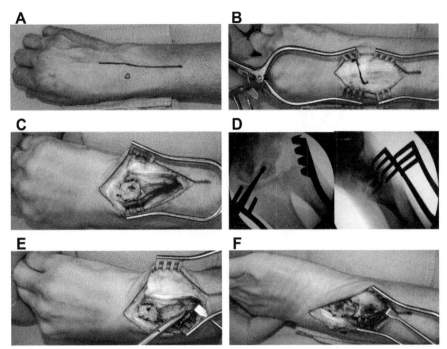

Fig. 2. Transfer of vascularized 4,5 extracompartmental artery bone flap to the lunate. (*A*) Dorsal skin incision. (*B*) Step-cut in extensor retinaculum during exposure of the dorsal wrist. (*C*) Exposure of the lunate (outlined) with core of necrotic bone removed. (*D*) Intraoperative fluoroscopic images of lunate. (*E*) Exposure and transection of posterior division of anterior interosseous artery with tenotomy scissors during flap harvest. (*F*) Pedicled flap harvest and transposition into lunate defect.

bone is probed for areas of necrosis. If the area of soft, necrotic bone is minimal, then a joint leveling procedure is performed without any further revascularization procedure. If there is necrotic bone, it is excised until a shell of cartilage and healthy cancellous bone remains (**Fig. 2**C, D). The articular shell can be gently expanded from the inside out if there is some collapse but preserved cartilage.

Once the size of the defect in the lunate has been measured, we proceed with the 4,5 ECA flap harvest (see **Fig. 2**B). The fifth ECA is identified on the floor of its extensor compartment while retracting the extensor digiti minimi tendon. The artery with its venae comitantes are traced proximally to their origin at the posterior division of the AIA. The fourth ECA branch is then identified and followed distally to its nutrient branches to the distal radius, usually 1-cm proximal to the articular surface (**Fig. 2**E). Osteotomes are then used to harvest a corticocancellous graft of the appropriate size. Once the bone flap has been elevated from the distal radius, the posterior branch of the AIA is ligated just proximal to where it divides into the fourth and fifth ECA. Retrograde arterial flow is obtained through the larger fifth ECA, with antegrade flow through the fourth ECA. The bone flap is mobilized and inset into

the lunate defect (**Fig. 2**F). The flap is oriented in such a way that the cortical surface is dorsal and can serve as a strut.

Favorable outcomes have been reported using vascularized distal radius pedicled flaps in Lichtman stage II-IIIB disease. Moran and colleagues[52] followed 26 patients for a mean of 31 months and found that the 4,5 ECA flap provided reliable improvement in pain, patient-reported outcomes, and grip strength (from 50% to 89% of the unaffected side), with preserved range of motion. Radiographic outcomes were also favorable, as 77% of patients showed no further evidence of lunate collapse, and 71% of patients with follow-up MRIs showed evidence of revascularization. In a recent study, Hegazy and colleagues[53] evaluated 21 patients with Lichtman stage II disease and 24 patients with stage IIIA disease. For each group, roughly half of the patients underwent revascularization with a 4,5 ECA flap and lunate unloading with a capitate shortening osteotomy, whereas the other half underwent lunate unloading only. Although outcomes were equivalent for the 2 procedures in patients with stage II disease, patients with stage IIIA disease who underwent the combined treatment had significantly better range of motion, grip strength, and patient-reported

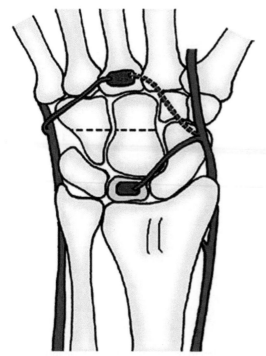

Fig. 3. Simplified schematic of third metacarpal base vascularized flap transfer. The pedicle is based on a dorsal metacarpal artery branch from the radial artery and the corticocancellous flap is set into the defect in the necrotic lunate. (*From* Waitayawinyu T, Chin SH, Luria S, Trumble TE. Capitate shortening osteotomy with vascularized bone grafting for the treatment of Kienböck disease in the ulnar positive wrist. J Hand Surg Am. 2008;33(8):1270; with permission).

outcomes. In these patients, the rate of failure for the combined procedure was 8%, compared with 28% when using the capitate-shortening osteotomy alone. Unfortunately, there remains a paucity of comparative outcomes in the literature to guide management.

Pedicled Proximal Metacarpal Flaps

Pedicled vascularized bone flaps from the metacarpal bases capitalize on the redundant circulation on the dorsum of the hand. The basal metacarpal arch gives off branches to the metacarpal bases via dorsal metacarpal arteries.[54,55] The arteries to the first and second metacarpal bases are more reliably present than branches to the ulnar metacarpals (**Fig. 3**). We use flaps based on the second or third dorsal metacarpal arteries in patients with ulnar positive wrists in conjunction with a capitate shortening osteotomy or capitohamate fusion for joint unloading (**Fig. 4**A). Because the bone harvest and the easier capitate shortening procedure are within the same wrist incision,

this technique has become our preferred procedure in unloading the lunate and in revascularizing this bone.

Under a regional block with tourniquet control, we use a longitudinal midline incision made dorsally.[56] Extensor pollicis longus is transposed from the third extensor compartment and a capsulotomy is made between the second and fourth compartments. The lunate is inspected, debrided of necrotic bone, and contoured as described earlier. The size of the bone defect is measured. We typically perform a capitate shortening osteotomy before harvesting the bone graft (**Fig. 4**B). Often the capitate and hamate are strongly tethered and need to be shortened to maintain congruity between the proximal and distal carpal rows. The bone fragments can be fused using K-wires or a compression screw in the capitate. The corticocancellous graft from the base of the metacarpal is then harvested and inset (**Fig. 4**C). The second and third dorsal metacarpal artery pedicles have enough excursion from the basal metacarpal arch to be used as retrograde flow vascularized flaps to the lunate.

Waitayawinyu and colleagues[24] studied 14 patients with ulnar positive wrists and Lichtman stage II-IIIA disease who underwent concomitant capitate-shortening procedures and lunate revascularization with a pedicled flap from the third metacarpal base. With a follow-up of 26 to 65 months, they demonstrated significant improvements in grip strength and satisfaction scores, while wrist range of motion was maintained despite the partial fusion procedure. Thirteen patients returned to their previous occupation and 12 returned to their previous level of function. Studies have obtained similar findings with follow-up of 10 years or more, showing equivalent results to distal radius pedicled flaps.[49,57]

Free Femoral Trochlea Flaps

The most extensively studied osseocartilaginous transfer technique uses a free vascularized flap from the medial femoral trochlea (MFT).[58,59] Its advent has greatly expanded the indications for lunate revascularization by transplanting vascularized bone together with healthy articular cartilage. This technique is indicated for lunate bone loss together with disruption of its proximal articular surface, and can be used in conjunction with unloading procedures or partial wrist fusions. It offers a much needed alternative to wrist salvage for young patients with advanced Kienböck disease. For patients older than 50 years, a proximal row carpectomy is still our preferred option given the ease of bone removal and the relative longevity

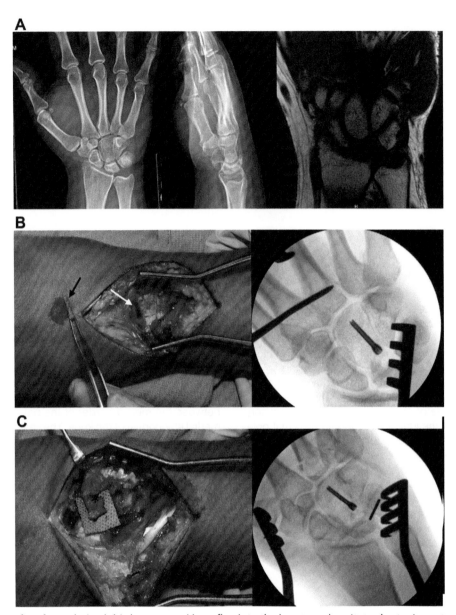

Fig. 4. Transfer of vascularized third metacarpal base flap into the lunate and capitate-shortening osteotomy. (*A*) Radiographs and MRI of a patient with Kienböck disease and an ulnar neutral wrist. (*B*) Intraoperative photograph of capitate osteotomy (*white arrow*) with removal of a wedge of bone (*black arrow*) and fluoroscopic image of fixation with a compression screw. (*C*) Intraoperative photograph of metacarpal flap harvest on its pedicle (*) and fluoroscopic image of fixation to the lunate with a Kirschner wire.

of this procedure. The main drawback of the free vascularized bone flap is that it is technically challenging, requiring consideration of the shape of the articular contour to be restored as well as microsurgical expertise. Donor site morbidity in harvesting a flap from the knee and the prolonged recovery process should be weighed carefully when considering the risks and benefits of surgery with the patient.[60–62] Salvage procedures such as proximal row carpectomy, wrist fusion, or total

wrist arthroplasty may still be necessary at a later time if intractable pain occurs persists despite attempting to preserve the lunate.

The MFT flap requires an understanding of the local anatomy in the knee, which has been well described in the literature. The flap is based on branches of the dorsal geniculate artery (DGA) from the superficial femoral artery.[63] Notable branches from the DGA include the saphenous artery branch and dorsal cutaneous branch

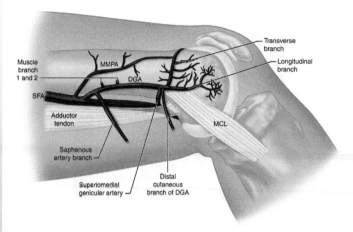

Fig. 5. Schematic of vascular anatomy of the medial femoral condyle. DGA, descending genicular artery; MCL, medial collateral ligament; MMPA, medial metaphyseal periosteal artery; SFA, superficial femoral artery. (*From* Iorio ML, Masden DL, Higgins JP. Cutaneous angiosome territory of the medial femoral condyle osteocutaneous flap. J Hand Surg Am. 2012;37(5):1034; with permission)

proximally, which can be used to elevate a skin paddle together with the osteochondral flap. Distally, the DGA gives off a transverse branch and a longitudinal branch that travel along the periosteum to the medial femoral condyle (**Fig. 5**). These have terminal branches that provide blood flow to the subchondral surface. Owing to the articular shape of the femoral condyle at the end points for these branches, the transverse branch is the pedicle of choice for osteochondral reconstruction of the lunate or scaphoid proximal pole, whereas the longitudinal branch is typically used when harvesting a vascularized bone flap without a chondral segment (ie, reconstruction of scaphoid waist nonunions).[58,64] The pedicle can be harvested as proximally as the origin of the DGA, resulting in a length of up to 8 cm.

When preparing to use the MFT flap for Kienböck disease, we perform an open or arthroscopic examination of the wrist to confirm the erosion of proximal lunate articular cartilage and

subchondral bone loss. We also examine the lunocapitate articulation to ensure that these cartilage surfaces are preserved (**Fig. 7**A, B). During the procedure, 2 teams work simultaneously in the operating room. The patient is positioned supine under general anesthesia supplemented by regional blocks. The affected arm and ipsilateral leg are exsanguinated and tourniquets are inflated. A curving longitudinal incision is centered midway between the medial border of the patella and the medial epicondyle of the knee. The vastus medialis is elevated anteriorly in the subfascial plane. This brings the DGA into view, which is followed along the periosteum to the medial knee. The transverse branch is identified by its anteriorly directed path to the articular surface of the MFT (**Fig. 6**A).

At the same time, the second team exposes the lunate through a midline dorsal exposure, as discussed earlier. Subtotal resection of the necrotic lunate and proximal articular cartilage is performed. The size of the defect in the lunate is

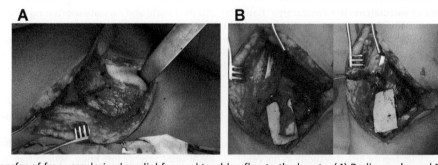

Fig. 6. Transfer of free vascularized medial femoral trochlea flap to the lunate. (*A*) Radiographs and MRI of a patient with Kienböck disease and disruption of the proximal lunate articulation. (*B*) Intraoperative photograph of preserved capitatolunate joint. (*C*) Detached radial artery branch to the first dorsal interosseous (*white arrow*) and adjacent lunate defect outlined. (*D*) Microscopic anastomosis of transverse branch of dorsal geniculate artery (***) and its 2 venae comitantes to the recipient vessels. (*E*) Intraoperative fluoroscopic image after inset of the flap into the lunate defect.

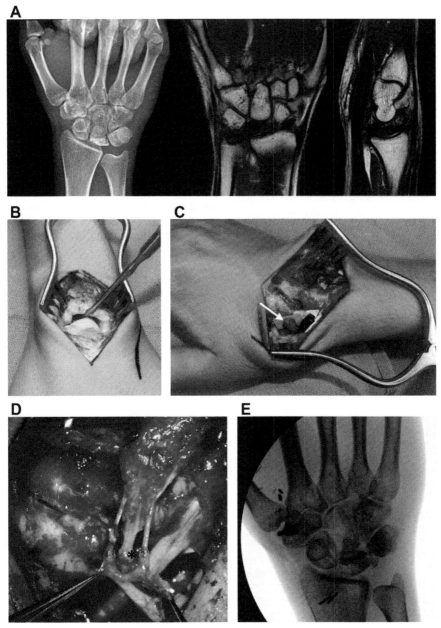

Fig. 7. Harvest of free vascularized medial femoral trochlea osseocartilaginous flap. (*A*) Photograph of the exposed medial femoral condyle, including the transverse branch (*) of the descending genicular artery and the outlined flap donor site. (*B*) Elevation of the osseocartilaginous flap on its pedicle.

measured in 3 dimensions and a marker is used to draw a templated flap onto the articular surface of the MFT. The osseocartilaginous flap and its pedicle, including the transverse arterial branch of the DGA and its 2 venae comitantes, are then harvested (**Fig. 6**B). We typically harvest as much of the DGA as possible in case additional length is needed. We inset the flap in the lunate defect and, under the microscope, perform an end-to-end arterial anastomosis with a terminal branch of the radial artery to the first dorsal interosseous muscle (**Fig. 7**C–E). We also perform anastomoses of the 2 venae comitantes to terminal branches of the cephalic vein. These vessels can all be accessed through the same dorsal incision used to expose the lunate. Finally, we use 1 or 2 screws to obtain fixation between the distal pole of the lunate and the MFT flap.

Several studies have demonstrated successful outcomes of lunate revascularization with the free

MFT flap. In a series of 16 patients with Lichtman stage II-IIIB disease followed for 12 to 34 months, Bürger and colleagues[58] showed radiographic healing and improved pain in all but 1 patient. Grip strength was improved to 85% of the contralateral side and range of motion was preserved. Lichtman stage remained stable in 10 patients, improved in 4, and worsened in 2. In a recent study, 23 patients with Lichtman stage IIIA-C Kienböck disease underwent lunate revascularization with a free osseocartilaginous flap harvested from the lateral femoral trochlea (LFT).[65] The pedicle of this flap is based on the superior lateral geniculate artery located under the iliotibial band.[66] Using this novel flap, Windhofer and colleagues[65] were able to closely match the contour of the articular defect in the lunate. At a mean follow-up of 34 months, 18 of 23 grafts were consolidated and patients demonstrated improved patient-reported outcomes with preserved range of motion, grip and pinch strength. Lichtman stage remained stable or improved in all but 2 patients. Although the specific indications for the LFT flap remain to be determined, the elucidation of alternative articular surfaces amenable to free flap harvest promises to revolutionize our approach to lunate revascularization in the future.

CLINICS CARE POINTS: KEY TECHNICAL PEARLS AND PITFALLS

- Always assess the bone quality and cartilage of the lunate before proceeding with a revascularization procedure, with either an open or arthroscopic technique.

- Evaluation of the ulnar variance can be helpful in deciding on the optimal pedicled bone flap based on the location of additional procedures for lunate unloading.

- Using a dorsal distal radius flap based on the fourth and fifth ECAs maximizes excursion compared with flaps based on the fourth ECA alone.

- The second metacarpal base has a larger and more consistent dorsal metacarpal artery than the third metacarpal base. However, the flap site with enough excursion to reach the lunate should be selected.

- The free MFT flap should be based on the transverse branch of the DGA. The articular site supplied by this branch closely approximates the contour of the proximal lunate articulation.

SUMMARY

Although the concept of lunate revascularization is not new, it has emerged as the promising next frontier in the treatment of Kienböck disease over the past decade. Of the many treatment options for this debilitating and still poorly understood disorder, revascularization procedures provide the most direct mechanism for reversing the pathologic process of osteonecrosis and restoring functional anatomy. Numerous pedicled bone flaps provide a reliable treatment for early disease and free vascularized flaps can be used in lieu of salvage operations for more advanced cases involving cartilage loss. The discovery of alternative free osseocartilaginous flap options may even further expand the indications for this technique in the future. Although recently developed techniques are promising, there is still a paucity of published research on their outcomes, and larger comparative studies are needed. Given the rarity of Kienböck disease, what is lacking in the literature to date is a prospective, collaborative, multicenter approach to determining the optimal surgical treatments for different stages of disease.

REFERENCES

1. Wagner JP, Chung KC. A historical report on Robert Kienböck (1871-1953) and Kienböck's Disease. J Hand Surg Am 2005;30(6):1117–21.
2. Golay SK, Rust P, Ring D. The Radiological Prevalence of Incidental Kienböck Disease. Arch Bone Jt Surg 2016;4(3):220–3.
3. van Leeuwen WF, Janssen SJ, ter Meulen DP, et al. What is the radiographic prevalence of incidental Kienböck Disease? Clin Orthop Relat Res 2016; 474(3):808–13.
4. Lluch A, Garcia-Elias M. Etiology of Kienböck disease. Tech Hand Up Extrem Surg 2011;15(1):33–7.
5. Rioux-Forker D, Shin AY. Osteonecrosis of the Lunate: Kienböck Disease. J Am Acad Orthop Surg 2020;28(14):570–84.
6. Schuind F, Eslami S, Ledoux P. Kienbock's disease. J Bone Joint Surg Br 2008;90(2):133–9.
7. Keith PP, Nuttall D, Trail I. Long-term outcome of nonsurgically managed Kienböck's disease. J Hand Surg Am 2004;29(1):63–7.
8. van Leeuwen WF, Tarabochia MA, Schuurman AH, et al. Risk factors of lunate collapse in Kienböck Disease. J Hand Surg Am 2017;42(11):883–8.e1.
9. Kristensen SS, Thomassen E, Christensen F. Kienböck's disease–late results by non-surgical treatment. A follow-up study. J Hand Surg Br 1986; 11(3):422–5.
10. Stahl S, Hentschel PJ, Held M, et al. Characteristic features and natural evolution of Kienböck's

disease: five years' results of a prospective case series and retrospective case series of 106 patients. J Plast Reconstr Aesthet Surg 2014;67(10):1415–26.

11. van Leeuwen WF, Janssen SJ, Ring D. Radiographic Progression of Kienböck Disease: radial shortening versus no surgery. J Hand Surg Am 2016;41(6): 681–8.

12. Persson M. Causal treatment of lunatomalacia; further experiences of operative ulna lengthening. Acta Chir Scand 1950;100(6):531–44.

13. Stahl S, Lotter O, Santos Stahl A, et al. 100 years after Kienböck's description: review of the etiology of Kienböck's disease from a historical perspective]. Orthopade 2012;41(1):66–72.

14. Durbin FC. The early changes of Kienböck's disease of the carpal lunate bone. Proc R Soc Med 1951; 44(6):482–8.

15. Gelberman RH, Bauman TD, Menon J, et al. The vascularity of the lunate bone and Kienböck's disease. J Hand Surg Am 1980;5(3):272–8.

16. Lee ML. The intraosseus arterial pattern of the carpal lunate bone and its relation to avascular necrosis. Acta Orthop Scand 1963;33:43–55.

17. Jensen CH. Intraosseous pressure in Kienböck's disease. J Hand Surg Am 1993;18(2):355–9.

18. Schiltenwolf M, Martini AK, Mau HC, et al. Further investigations of the intraosseous pressure characteristics in necrotic lunates (Kienböck's disease). J Hand Surg Am 1996;21(5):754–8.

19. Watson HK, Guidera PM. Aetiology of Kienböck's disease. J Hand Surg Br 1997;22(1):5–7.

20. Freedman DM, Botte MJ, Gelberman RH. Vascularity of the carpus. Clin Orthop Relat Res 2001; 383:47–59.

21. Gellman H, Botte MJ, Shankwiler J, et al. Arterial patterns of the deep and superficial palmar arches. Clin Orthop Relat Res 2001;383:41–6.

22. Sheetz KK, Bishop AT, Berger RA. The arterial blood supply of the distal radius and ulna and its potential use in vascularized pedicled bone grafts. J Hand Surg Am 1995;20(6):902–14.

23. Elhassan BT, Shin AY. Vascularized bone grafting for treatment of Kienböck's disease. J Hand Surg Am 2009;34(1):146–54.

24. Waitayawinyu T, Chin SH, Luria S, et al. Capitate shortening osteotomy with vascularized bone grafting for the treatment of Kienböck's disease in the ulnar positive wrist. J Hand Surg Am 2008;33(8): 1267–73.

25. Higgins JP, Bürger HK. Medial femoral trochlea osteochondral flap: applications for scaphoid and lunate reconstruction. Clin Plast Surg 2020;47(4): 491–9.

26. Kenzora JE, Glimcher MJ. Pathogenesis of idiopathic osteonecrosis: the ubiquitous crescent sign. Orthop Clin North Am 1985;16(4):681–96.

27. Enneking WF, Eady JL, Burchardt H. Autogenous cortical bone grafts in the reconstruction of segmental skeletal defects. J Bone Joint Surg Am 1980;62(7):1039–58.

28. Han CS, Wood MB, Bishop AT, et al. Vascularized bone transfer. J Bone Joint Surg Am 1992;74(10): 1441–9.

29. Moran SL, Shin AY. Vascularized bone grafting for the treatment of carpal pathology. Orthop Clin North Am 2007;38(1):73–85.

30. Sunagawa T, Bishop AT, Muramatsu K. Role of conventional and vascularized bone grafts in scaphoid nonunion with avascular necrosis: a canine experimental study. J Hand Surg Am 2000;25(5):849–59.

31. Tu YK, Bishop AT, Kato T, et al. Experimental carpal reverse-flow pedicle vascularized bone grafts. Part II: bone blood flow measurement by radioactive-labeled microspheres in a canine model. J Hand Surg Am 2000;25(1):46–54.

32. Hori Y, Tamai S, Okuda H, et al. Blood vessel transplantation to bone. J Hand Surg Am 1979;4(1): 23–33.

33. Higgins JP, Borumandi F, Bürger HK, et al. Nonvascularized cartilage grafts versus vascularized cartilage flaps: comparison of cartilage quality 6 months after transfer. J Hand Surg Am 2018;43(2): 188.e1–8.

34. Kennedy C, Abrams R. In Brief: The Lichtman Classification for Kienböck Disease. Clin Orthop Relat Res 2019;477(6):1516–20.

35. Murphey MD, Foreman KL, Klassen-Fischer MK, et al. From the radiologic pathology archives imaging of osteonecrosis: radiologic-pathologic correlation. Radiographics 2014;34(4):1003–28.

36. Stevens K, Tao C, Lee SU, et al. Subchondral fractures in osteonecrosis of the femoral head: comparison of radiography, CT, and MR imaging. Am J Roentgenol 2003;180(2):363–8.

37. Rhee PC, Jones DB, Moran SL, et al. The effect of lunate morphology in Kienböck disease. J Hand Surg Am 2015;40(4):738–44.

38. Mohan A, Knight R, Ismail H, et al. Radiographic and computed tomography correlation of kienbock's disease: is there a need to revisit staging with improved imaging? J Wrist Surg 2020;9(1):39–43.

39. Arnaiz J, Piedra T, Cerezal L, et al. Imaging of Kienböck disease. Am J Roentgenol 2014;203(1):131–9.

40. Large TM, Adams MR, Loeffler BJ, et al. Posttraumatic avascular necrosis after proximal femur, proximal humerus, talar neck, and scaphoid fractures. J Am Acad Orthop Surg 2019;27(21):794–805.

41. Goldfarb CA, Hsu J, Gelberman RH, et al. The Lichtman classification for Kienböck's disease: an assessment of reliability. J Hand Surg Am 2003; 28(1):74–80.

42. Shin M, Tatebe M, Hirata H, et al. Reliability of Lichtman's classification for Kienböck's disease in 99 subjects. Hand Surg 2011;16(1):15–8.

43. MacLean SBM, Kantar K, Bain GI, et al. The Role of wrist arthroscopy in kienbock disease. Hand Clin 2017;33(4):727–34.

44. Bain GI, Begg M. Arthroscopic assessment and classification of Kienbock's disease. Tech Hand Up Extrem Surg 2006;10(1):8–13.

45. Bain GI, MacLean SB, Tse WL, et al. Kienböck disease and arthroscopy: assessment, classification, and treatment. J Wrist Surg 2016;5(4):255–60.

46. Bain GI, MacLean SB, Yeo CJ, et al. The etiology and pathogenesis of kienböck disease. J Wrist Surg 2016;5(4):248–54.

47. Shin AY, Bishop AT. Pedicled vascularized bone grafts for disorders of the carpus: scaphoid nonunion and Kienbock's disease. J Am Acad Orthop Surg 2002;10(3):210–6.

48. Zaidemberg C, Siebert JW, Angrigiani C. A new vascularized bone graft for scaphoid nonunion. J Hand Surg Am 1991;16(3):474–8.

49. Fujiwara H, Oda R, Morisaki S, et al. Long-term results of vascularized bone graft for stage III Kienböck disease. J Hand Surg Am 2013;38(5):904–8.

50. Daecke W, Lorenz S, Wieloch P, et al. Lunate resection and vascularized Os pisiform transfer in Kienböck's Disease: an average of 10 years of follow-up study after Saffar's procedure. J Hand Surg Am 2005;30(4):677–84.

51. Berger RA, Bishop AT, Bettinger PC. New dorsal capsulotomy for the surgical exposure of the wrist. Ann Plast Surg 1995;35(1):54–9.

52. Moran SL, Cooney WP, Berger RA, et al. The use of the 4 + 5 extensor compartmental vascularized bone graft for the treatment of Kienböck's disease. J Hand Surg Am 2005;30(1):50–8.

53. Hegazy G, Seddik M, Massoud AH, et al. Capitate shortening osteotomy with or without vascularized bone grafting for the treatment of early stages of Kienböck's disease. Int Orthop 2021;45(10):2635–41.

54. Bermel C, Saalabian AA, Horch RE, et al. Vascularization of the dorsal base of the second metacarpal bone: an anatomical study using C-arm cone beam computed tomography. Plast Reconstr Surg 2014;134(1):72e–80e.

55. Dauphin N, Casoli V. The dorsal metacarpal arteries: anatomical study. Feasibility of pedicled metacarpal bone flaps. J Hand Surg Eur 2011;36(9):787–94.

56. Grant DW, Chung KC. Chapter 31: Procedures for Avascular Necrosis of the Lunate (Kienböck Disease). In: Chung KC, editor. Operative techniques: hand and wrist surgery. 4th edition. Elsevier; 2021. p. 194–210.

57. Nakagawa M, Omokawa S, Kira T, et al. Vascularized bone grafts from the dorsal wrist for the treatment of kienböck disease. J Wrist Surg 2016;5(2):98–104.

58. Bürger HK, Windhofer C, Gaggl AJ, et al. Vascularized medial femoral trochlea osteochondral flap reconstruction of advanced Kienböck disease. J Hand Surg Am 2014;39(7):1313–22.

59. Van Handel AC, Lynch LM, Daruwalla JH, et al. Medial femoral trochlea flap reconstruction versus proximal row carpectomy for Kienböck's disease: a morphometric comparison. J Hand Surg Eur 2021;46(10):1042–8.

60. Pet MA, Assi PE, Giladi AM, et al. Preliminary clinical, radiographic, and patient-reported outcomes of the medial femoral trochlea osteochondral free flap for lunate reconstruction in advanced kienböck disease. J Hand Surg Am 2020;45(8):774.e1–8.

61. Pet MA, Assi PE, Yousaf IS, et al. Outcomes of the medial femoral trochlea osteochondral free flap for proximal scaphoid reconstruction. J Hand Surg Am 2020;45(4):317–26.e3.

62. Pet MA, Higgins JP. Long-term outcomes of vascularized trochlear flaps for scaphoid proximal pole reconstruction. Hand Clin 2019;35(3):345–52.

63. Iorio ML, Masden DL, Higgins JP. Cutaneous angiosome territory of the medial femoral condyle osteocutaneous flap. J Hand Surg Am 2012;37(5):1033–41.

64. Bürger HK, Windhofer C, Gaggl AJ, et al. Vascularized medial femoral trochlea osteocartilaginous flap reconstruction of proximal pole scaphoid nonunions. J Hand Surg Am 2013;38(4):690–700.

65. Windhofer CM, Anoshina M, Ivusits P, et al. The free vascularized lateral femoral trochlea osteochondral graft: a reliable alternative for Stage III Kienböck's disease. J Hand Surg Eur 2021;46(10):1032–41.

66. Morsy M, Sur YJ, Akdag O, et al. Anatomic and high-resolution computed tomographic angiography study of the lateral femoral condyle flap: implications for surgical dissection. J Plast Reconstr Aesthet Surg 2018;71(1):33–43.

Wrist Salvage Procedures for the Treatment of Kienbock's Disease

Jeremy A. Adler, MD[1], Megan Conti Mica, MD*, Cathleen Cahill, MD[2]

KEYWORDS

- Kienbock's disease • Avascular necrosis of lunate • Wrist salvage procedures
- Total wrist arthroplasty • Proximal row carpectomy

KEY POINTS

- Etiology of Kienbock's disease is considered to be multifactorial.
- Treatment options vary based on the stage of disease.
- In cases of advanced Kienbock's disease, wrist salvage procedures are the preferred treatment option.
- The most common surgical options include PRC and total wrist arthrodesis and less commonly TWA.

INTRODUCTION

Kienbock's disease, or avascular necrosis of the lunate, is a chronic progressive degenerative condition that can eventually lead to pancarpal arthritis with loss of function, grip strength, and pain.[1] In 1910, an Australian radiologist by the name of Robert Kienbock first described this disease radiographically as osteomalacia of the lunate. He noted radiographic changes of the proximal portion of the lunate, specifically at the radiolunate junction and suggested that these changes were secondary to the rupture of ligaments and blood vessels. This, he believed, caused an osseous nutritional deficiency that in late cases could be treated by lunate excision.[2] Currently, there exist a variety of operative treatments for the disease in its various stages. In this article, we will address the more advanced stages of Kienbock's disease with attention to options for wrist salvage.

Etiology

The etiology of Kienbock's disease is likely multifactorial, including vascular and skeletal anatomic variations in combination with microtrauma or repetitive loading.[3] There is no confirmed genetic predisposition to Kienbock's disease.

Blood supply to the lunate is considered to be a contributing factor to the development of Kienbock's disease. In one study examining the arterial supply of the lunate, the majority (65%) of patients had dual flow via both dorsal and palmar arteries with an intraosseous anastomosis. Other patterns of arterial supply included dual extraosseous vascularity (7.5%) and single vessel blood supply (26%). Single vessel blood supply with minimal anastomosis may predispose certain patients to lunate osteonecrosis in the setting of isolated or repetitive trauma.[4] However, this single vessel anatomic variant is likely only one of many contributing factors, as Gelberman and colleagues reported 80% of lunates had palmar and dorsal blood supply.[2] Increased intraosseous pressure of the lunate may also play a role in lunate necrosis.[5] Ulnar negative variance has also been a proposed etiology of Kienbock's disease. However, D'Hoore and colleagues compared 125 normal wrists to 52 wrists with Kienbock's disease and found no statically significant difference in ulnar variance between the two groups.[6]

UChicago Medicine and Biological Sciences, Chicago, IL 60637, USA
[1] Present address: 65 East Monroe Street, Apartment 4007, Chicago, IL 60603.
[2] Present address: 2400 North Lakeview Avenue, Apartment 2301, Chicago, IL 60614.
* Corresponding author. 5841 South Maryland Avenue, MC3079, Chicago, IL 60637.
E-mail address: mcontimica@bsd.uchicago.edu

Hand Clin 38 (2022) 447–459
https://doi.org/10.1016/j.hcl.2022.03.012

Kienbock's disease appears to be more common in laborers; however, there is no proven association between a single traumatic event and the development of osteonecrosis of the lunate.[7] Perilunate dislocation may cause increased focal radiodensity of the lunate although there is no proven association with this radiographic finding and the carpal collapse observed in Kienbock's disease.[7,8] The exact etiology of Kienbock's disease continues to be a controversial topic and is likely associated with an interplay of osseous and vascular insults in the setting of microtrauma.

Presentation

Patients with Kienbock's present with symptoms that vary and radiographic findings that do not always correlate with the clinical presentation.[3] This condition is most common in men aged 20 to 40 years. Most cases are unilateral and involve the dominant hand. Although most cases occur in healthy individuals, some case reports suggest an association with systemic lupus erythematosus (SLE), sickle cell anemia, scleroderma, rheumatoid arthritis, dermatomyositis, and gout.[3,9–11] Dorsal wrist tenderness and swelling are common early manifestations.[12] As the disease progresses, pain and wrist motion begin to interfere with daily activities, and this is the period where many patients first present for a formal evaluation. In cases of advanced disease, patients may report pain at rest, decreased grip strength, and severely limited range of motion.

Diagnostic Imaging

Most patients presenting with dorsal wrist pain undergo preliminary radiographs including posteroanterior, lateral, and oblique views of the wrist. Radiographically, Kienbock's disease is characterized based on the extent of sclerosis and trabecular collapse of the lunate. Initially disease will not be detected on radiographs alone and can only be detected on MRI. As the disease progresses, radiographs may show sclerosis of the lunate with eventual collapse, with eventual local involvement of the scaphoid and further involvement of the remaining carpus in late stages. The loss of carpal height, proximal migration of the capitate, and hyperflexion of the scaphoid are important for classification and for surgical planning. As mentioned previously, MRI is the gold standard imaging study for the detection of lunate avascular necrosis in cases where the lunate collapse is not yet apparent on plain radiographs. In later stages, CT is used to characterize the extent of arthritis involving neighboring carpal bones and can aid in preoperative planning.

Staging

Early Kienbock's disease can present radiographically with sclerosis of the lunate and can progress to complete central column collapse. Abnormal carpal motion and deformity may result in degenerative changes throughout the carpal and radiocarpal joints. First described in 1977, Lichtman's classification is commonly used to detail disease progression and to stage disease and compare outcomes[13] (Fig. 1).

The progression of Kienbock's disease starts with the isolated proximal lunate disease to sclerosis and collapse of the lunate and lastly to radiocarpal degenerative changes.[14] According to the Lichtman classification system, Stage I presents with normal radiographs or possible linear fractures of the lunate, and diagnosis can often only be made with MRI demonstrating avascular necrosis (Fig. 2). At this stage, patients often report intermittent wrist pain.[1] Stage II demonstrates radiodensity of the lunate, indicating sclerosis but without collapse. Clinically, patients report increased pain and swelling and may or may not develop wrist stiffness.[1] Stage IIIA consists of lunate collapse and fragmentation, in addition to proximal migration of the capitate (Fig. 3) creating loss of carpal height without associated carpal malalignment.

In Stage IIIB, in addition to findings seen in IIIA, the scaphoid flexes (Fig. 4) and radiographs demonstrate an increased radioscaphoid angle of more than 60°.[15] Typically, by Stage III, patients report increased pain and decreased grip strength.[1] Central column collapse and proximal row instability can eventually progress to radial column collapse. The degeneration of the radial column causes progression to Stage IV.[16] Stage IV includes IIIB findings with generalized degenerative changes throughout the midcarpal joints, radiocarpal joint, or both.[3]

Treatment

Treatment can be guided by using the Lichtman classification. Treatment of Lichtman Stages I, II, and IIIA is primarily focused on preserving lunate morphology, vascularity, and wrist biomechanics, ranging from immobilization to a variety of osteotomies, vascularized bone grafting, metaphyseal core decompression, and intercarpal fusions.[17] In Stage IIIB, limited intercarpal fusion and proximal row carpectomy (PRC) can be performed. This bypasses the diseased central column.[18]

Once the radioscaphoid articulation becomes compromised in Stage IV, the wrist can no longer be reconstructed and salvage procedures are

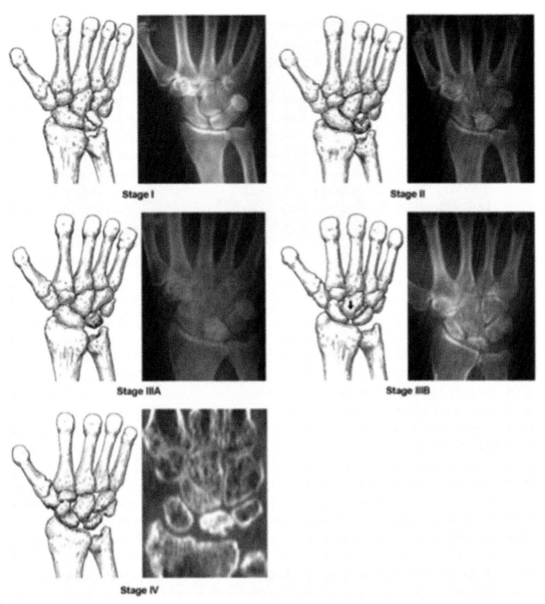

Fig. 1. Images represent the progressive stages of Kienbock disease described in the Lichtman classification. Stage I consists of normal radiographs with decreased T1 signal consistent with AVN. Stage 2 demonstrates lunate sclerosis. Stage IIIA presents with lunate collapse, while IIIB demonstrates lunate and carpal collapse with scaphoid rotation. Stage IV consists of radial and central column collapse with associated pancarpal arthritis. (*From* Allan CH, Joshi A, Lichtman DM. Kienbock's disease: diagnosis and treatment. *J Am Acad Orthop Surg*. 2001;9(2):128-136, with permission.)

required.[16] Interventions are directed at treating perilunate arthritis, with the goal of relieving pain and providing stability. Both motion sparing and motion sacrificing treatments are described and primarily include PRC, limited intercarpal fusion, total wrist fusion, or total wrist arthroplasty (TWA), with partial or total wrist denervation used as adjunctive or isolated procedures.[3]

Preoperative/Preprocedure Planning

A thorough history should be obtained in all patients, and preoperative range of motion, strength, and pain should be considered. Operative records from all prior surgical interventions, with attention to the intraoperative description of the articular cartilage of the capitate head and lunate fossa can be very helpful. PA and lateral radiographs

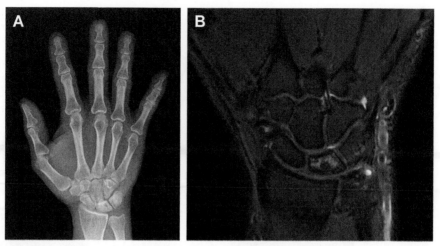

Fig. 2. PA radiograph (*A*) demonstrating sclerotic changes of the lunate without collapse. Coronal MRI (*B*) demonstrates avascular necrosis of the lunate.

are used to assess various anatomic factors including ulnar variance, radial inclination, carpal height, radioscaphoid angle, lunate size, and morphology. MRI is often used for staging and to detect the extent of osteonecrosis, whereas CT better characterizes the extent of articular surface collapse, the presence of fractures, and the available bone stock for potential arthrodesis or arthroplasty.[18] Even patients with advanced findings may still remain functional with only mild symptoms, therefore a trial of nonoperative treatment including bracing, anti-inflammatories, and corticosteroid injections are recommended regardless of the radiographic stage of initial presentation.

Prep and Patient Positioning

Patients may receive a peripheral nerve block with MAC anesthesia for surgery. Preoperative

antibiotic prophylaxis should be administered before incision. Patients are positioned in the supine position on the operating table with the affected arm abducted to 90° on a hand table. A tourniquet is placed proximally around the midbrachium to obtain a bloodless field. Standard sterile preparation and draping are performed.

Denervation

Denervation is a less intrusive and motion-sparing technique that treats patients with a primary complaint of wrist pain from degenerative arthritis secondary to fractures and dislocations of the carpus, ligamentous injuries, and Kienbock's disease.[19] This procedure interrupts specific afferent nerve fibers from the wrist joint.[19,20] Before the procedure, patients can go through a trial of relief by performing preoperative lidocaine nerve blocks

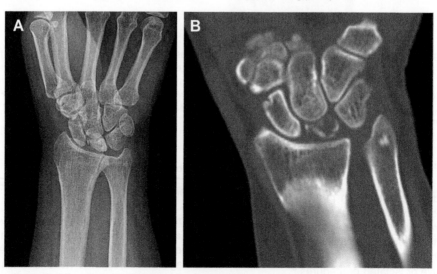

Fig. 3. PA radiograph (*A*) and coronal CT (*B*) demonstrate lunate fragmentation and collapse.

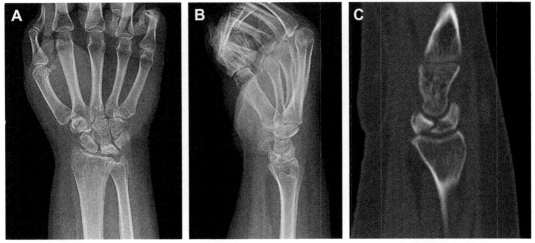

Fig. 4. PA and lateral radiographs (*A*, *B*) and sagittal CT (*C*) demonstrate lunate collapse with associated flexion of the scaphoid, seen in Stage IIIB Kienbock's.

of some or all of the sensory nerves around the wrist. Failure to relieve pain from preoperative nerve blocks can be considered a relative contra-indication to surgical denervation.[19] Typically, with Stage II Kienbock's disease, PIN denervation at the fourth dorsal compartment is performed at the time of additional surgery.[19] In Stages III and IV, complete wrist denervation has been described as an isolated procedure to provide pain relief in the arthritic wrist; however, potential drawbacks include multiple incisions, numbness, and the possibility of symptom recurrence.[21]

Surgical technique for wrist denervation
Wrist denervation is often performed under regional or general anesthesia as an outpatient procedure.

Partial denervation
- A 3–4 cm incision is made dorsally just proximal and ulnar to Lister's Tubercle
- Dissection is performed down to the floor of the fourth dorsal compartment and the posterior interosseous nerve (PIN) is identified, isolated, and a 1 cm portion of the nerve is excised
- A small incision is then made through the interosseous membrane (IOM)
- The AIN will be identified just deep to the IOM and typically ulnar to the PIN and a 1–2 mm section of nerve should be excised

Complete denervation
- AIN and PIN neurectomy are performed as outlined above.
- There is limited evidence supporting an ideal combination of nerve branches to target,

and given the extensive number of options, surgeons will often choose a subset of the nerves identified below for denervation.
- (1) posterior interosseus
- (2) articular branch of the first interosseus space
- (3) articular branch of the lateral antebrachial cutaneous
- (4) articular branch of the superficial radial nerve
- (5) palmar branch of the median nerve
- (6) articular fibers of the anterior interosseus nerve
- (7 and 8) perforating fibers of the deep branch of the ulnar nerve
- (9) dorsal branch of the ulnar nerve
- (10) articulating fibers of the posterior antebrachial cutaneous[19]

Postoperative protocol for wrist denervation
Following the procedure, the patient is placed in a soft dressing with a volar plaster splint for soft tissue rest. Full range of motion of the fingers and elbow are encouraged immediately following the procedure, and if performed in isolation, the splint can be discontinued at 2 weeks.[19]

Proximal row carpectomy
Proponents of PRC prefer this procedure as it is motion sparing, relatively simple, and leaves open the possibility for future wrist arthrodesis if indicated. After removal of the proximal row, the capitate head will articulate with the lunate fossa **(Fig. 5)** and therefore these articular surfaces must largely be void of any significant degenerative changes. Although severe arthritis of the capitate head is considered a contraindication to PRC,

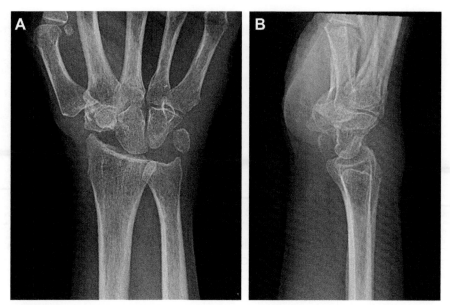

Fig. 5. PA and lateral radiographs obtained after proximal row carpectomy, demonstrating new articulation between the capitate head and lunate fossa of the radius. PA (*A*) and Lateral (*B*)

more mild changes are accepted by some. Interposition arthroplasty with dorsal wrist capsule or partial capitate resection can be performed at the time of PRC if mild arthritis is suspected.[22,23]

Surgical technique for *proximal row carpectomy*[24–26]

- Dorsal 7 to 8 cm longitudinal incision just ulnar to Lister's tubercle
- Dissection down to extensor retinaculum
- Elevate cutaneous radial and ulnar flaps taking care to protect sensory branches of the radial and ulnar nerves
- Identify extensor pollicis longus (EPL) coursing obliquely over the radial wrist extensors
- Open the retinaculum along the third dorsal compartments and retract EPL radially
- Make retinacular flaps to the second compartment radially and the fifth compartment ulnarly
- Identify the PIN in the fourth dorsal compartment
  ○ Resect a 1-cm segment of the PIN and cauterize the proximal stump
- Perform a standard or ligament sparing incision of the wrist capsule[27]
- Elevate capsule to visualize the scaphoid, lunate, and triquetrum
- Inspect articular surfaces of the lunate facet of the distal radius and capitate head to confirm the absence of significant chondromalacia
- Individually remove the scaphoid, lunate, and triquetrum, respectively, while reflecting the volar capsule and protecting the radioscaphocapitate (RSC) ligament off the scaphoid.
  ○ Kirshner wires can be placed to joystick the carpal bones and allow elevation of any soft tissue off the bone using a beaver blade, McGlamry elevator, or osteotome.
  ○ Injury to the RSC ligament can result in postoperative ulnar translation of the carpus
- Once the proximal carpal bones have been excised, confirm complete excision and appropriate seating of the capitate in the lunate fossa using fluoroscopic imaging
  ○ Confirm radial deviation does not cause impingement between the residual carpal bones and the radial styloid
  ○ If impingement is noted, a radial styloidectomy is indicated. The styloid should be skeletonized, and only 3 to 4 mm of bone should be excised using an osteotome. Any larger excision could create instability of the carpus by disrupting the styloid origin of the radioscaphoid capitate ligament.
- Closure
  ○ Approximate capsular flaps, retinaculum, and subcutaneous tissues with absorbable suture
  ○ Approximate skin using absorbable suture
  ○ Apply a well-padded volar resting splint

Postoperative protocol for proximal row carpectomy

Patients are discharged on the day of surgery with a volar resting splint with the MCP joints free. Digital motion is encouraged immediately after surgery. At the 2-week postoperative visit, the patient is transitioned to custom-fitted volar resting splint. After 4 weeks of immobilization, therapy with guided radiocarpal motion under the supervision of a hand therapist is initiated. By 6 weeks postoperatively, no immobilization is needed and strengthening should begin. Three months postoperatively, the patient can return to full unrestricted activities.[26]

Limited intercarpal arthrodesis

Partial wrist fusion is also a commonly described treatment option in advanced Kienbock's, most commonly in the form of STT or scaphocapitate (SC) intercarpal arthrodesis. The goal of surgery is to realign the scaphoid to stabilize the midcarpal joint, prevent further carpal collapse, and potentially slow the degenerative process. Biomechanical studies have suggested SC arthrodesis decreases radiolunate and lunocapitate forces with increased joint forces across the radioscaphoid joint.[28] Advocates may support this over PRC as it maintains carpal height and preserves the radioscaphoid articulation.[29] Some authors may favor STT fusion given prior reports of better motion postoperatively compared with SC fusion.[1] Sc arthrodesis provides a larger bony surface for fusion with only a single articulation, compared with STT with three separate smaller articulations. (Cross 2014). The ideal position of the scaphoid for an intercarpal arthrodesis is not clearly defined, but authors have recommended obtaining an intraoperative radioscaphoid angle of 30° to 60°.[29–31]

Surgical technique for limited intercarpal arthrodesis (scaphocapitate fusion)[29]

- Make longitudinal incision between second and fourth dorsal compartments
- Perform ligament sparing capsulotomy
- Expose SC articulation and remove all remaining articular cartilage
- If significant scaphoid flexion present, a 1.5 mm Kirschner wire can be inserted and used as a joystick to correct any palmar flexion deformity
- When satisfied with carpal position, provisionally insert a 1.5 mm Kirschner wire across the SC joint
- Bony compression/fixation can be performed using a headless cannulated compression screw(s), Kirschner wires, or plate construct
- In the setting of poor/limited bone quality, cancellous autograft may be used to supplement the arthrodesis
- Approximate capsule, subcutaneous tissues, and skin and apply a volar resting splint

Wrist arthrodesis

Total wrist fusion is a reliable but motion sacrificing surgery, which is potentially applicable to the management of nearly all of posttraumatic or degenerative wrist arthritis. The goal of surgery is to provide a stable wrist for power grip and provide adequate pain relief. Patients should have adequate shoulder, elbow, forearm, and digital motion to account for motion loss at the wrist. Other associated conditions such as carpal tunnel syndrome, DRUJ arthritis, and ulnocarpal impaction syndrome will not resolve with bony fusion alone, and patients should be counseled on this preoperatively.

Multiple techniques and fixation strategies have been described to obtain bony fusion between the carpus and radius. The most common fixation strategy for degenerative and post-traumatic arthritis is dorsal plating, while rod and pin fixation is a more commonly used for inflammatory arthritis or connective tissue disorders.[32] Autogenous cancellous bone graft from the iliac crest or the distal radial metaphysis can be incorporated into the fusion mass, particularly in those with poor bone stock seen on preoperative imaging. The benefits of rigid plate fixation include early postoperative rehabilitation and high fusion rate compared with other techniques.[32] Recommendations of wrist position at the time of fusion vary in the literature and should be based on the needs of the individual patient.[33–35]

Surgical technique for total wrist arthrodesis[32,36–38]

- Dorsal longitudinal incision over the third metacarpal base extending proximally, ulnar to Lister's tubercle
- Elevate cutaneous flaps taking care to protect cutaneous nerves and dorsal veins
- Open third dorsal compartment and retract EPL radially
- Elevate second and fourth dorsal compartments and perform a PIN neurectomy
- Sharply incise periosteum over dorsal third metacarpal, avoiding adjacent interosseous musculature
- Open the capsule with a T-shaped incision and expose the third carpometacarpal (CMC), capitolunate, and radiocarpal articulations
- Thoroughly assess the carpal articular surfaces
- Denude joint surfaces to bleeding cancellous bone
  - Radioscaphoid, radiolunate, scapholunate, SC, and lunocapitate articulations are commonly incorporated into fusion mass
  - Use a curette and a small round burr to remove all remaining cartilage and sclerotic bone

- Remove listers tubercle and decorticate dorsal surfaces of scaphoid, lunate, and capitate to create an even surface for plate application using osteotomes or a saw.
- Harvest autologous bone graft from the distal radial metaphysis using a cortical window 2 cm proximal to the distal radial articular surface
  ○ If a large bone defect or bone quality poor, consider obtaining iliac crest bone graft
  ○ Some surgeons prefer to begin this case with PRC, and in these cases, the excised carpal bones may be useful as a bone graft.
- Insert graft into prepared fusion sites
- Apply low profile contoured plate and confirm the position of plate and wrist using fluoroscopy before screw insertion
  ○ Place wrist in the desired position of fusion, generally 10° to 20° of extension, 5° to 10° of ulnar deviation
- Position plate as far proximally as possible on the metacarpal shaft to limit extensor tendon irritation
- Obtain bicortical fixation distally in the third metacarpal shaft, capitate, and radius and compress across the fusion mass
- Once the plate is securely placed with all screws aligned, confirm the final plate position using fluoroscopy
- Closure
  ○ Approximate capsule, and if needed a distally based slip from one of the wrist extensor tendons to aid in plate coverage
  ○ Approximate retinaculum, transpose EPL above extensor retinaculum
  ○ Approximate subcutaneous tissue
  ○ Approximate skin using nonabsorbable or absorbable sutures

Postoperative protocol for partial/complete wrist arthrodesis

Postoperatively patients are immobilized in a plaster splint or brace for a minimum of 6 to 8 weeks.[39] Once there is radiographic and clinical evidence of fusion, they can be transitioned out of immobilization and initiate supervised therapy to improve motion and strength. Generally time from surgery to union requires 8 to 12 weeks, and it is essential to encourage early active and passive digital motion to prevent stiffness and MCP joint extension contractures.[40]

Total Wrist Arthroplasty

Wrist arthroplasty has emerged as a motion-sparing surgical option for wrist arthritis and can allow patients to perform certain ADLs with less difficulty; however, it is still less commonly performed than arthrodesis. In 2008, the number of total wrist fusions was nearly 10 times the number of wrist arthroplasties performed.[41] Arthroplasty is more commonly used in lower demand elderly populations that is generally not the Kienbock's patient population.[17]

With newer generations of implants, it is increasingly being considered for younger patients with degenerative or posttraumatic arthritis who can accept postoperative restrictions such as heavy lifting, hyperextension loading, and high impact sports.[41] Fourth-generation implants are designed to improve stability, provide greater longevity, and minimize postoperative complications although there is limited long-term outcomes data.[41] TWA is contraindicated in those with compromise bone stock available for carpal fixation, soft tissue infection, intraarticular infection, or insufficient neuromuscular control.[42] Current implants only require screw fixation into the carpus and have a porous surface to improve bony ingrowth and support a noncemented technique.[41] This can theoretically improve durability and maintain bone stock making potential revision arthrodesis less challenging.[41]

Preoperative range of motion and the presence of any soft tissue contractures or instability should be considered as it may lead to limited motion or chronic instability following arthroplasty.[41] PA and lateral radiographs should be obtained to evaluate bony deformity and the presence of osteopenia and bony erosions. If the available bone stock is limited, autograft or cement can be considered to augment carpal component fixation to help prevent implant loosening. Radiographs should also be used preoperatively to template the carpal and radial components and to plan for the placement of radial and ulnar carpal screws.[42]

Surgical technique for TWA[41]

There are variations in technique depending on implant design and generation; however, basic principles include:

- Dorsal longitudinal incision in line with the third metacarpal, extending approximately 4 cm proximal to the radiocarpal joint
- Elevate cutaneous flaps taking care to protect cutaneous nerves and dorsal veins
- Sharply open ECU compartment and elevate retinaculum radially to the septum between the first and second compartments
  ○ Tip: The retinaculum can be opened in a step cut fashion to create radial/ulnar flaps to potentially augment capsular closure
- Perform ligament sparing capsulotomy
- Place wrist in hyperflexion, and prepare distal radius according to implant specific technique guide

○ Distal radius preparation can also be completed after the preparation of the carpus
- Cut and sequentially broach radius
  ○ Avoid injury/detachment of volar radiocarpal ligaments
- Trial radial components
- Prepare carpus using sagittal saw while protecting volar capsule (variable depending on implant used)
  ○ Can use Kirschner wires or Steinman pins to stabilize carpal bones before preparation
- Trial polyethylene carpal component and reduce wrist
- Assess range of motion, stability, and soft tissue balancing, except approximately 35° of flexion and extension
  ○ If the extension is limited, this may be secondary to a tight volar capsule, which can be remedied by excising additional radius.
  ○ If volar instability is encountered, consider the possibility of injury or detachment of the volar radiocarpal ligament complex.
- Insert final components using the press-fit technique
  ○ Avoid crossing fourth/fifth CMC joints during carpal fixation
  ○ Depending on bone stock and surgeon preference, cement may also be used
- Closure
  ○ Approximate capsule, retinaculum, and subcutaneous tissues
- If inadequate tissue for closure during terminal wrist flexion, pass distal extensor retinaculum underneath extensors to augment capsular closure
  ○ Apply bulky dressing

Postoperative protocol for wrist arthroplasty

Postoperative immobilization is generally continued for 2 to 4 weeks, but this is dependent on intraoperative assessment of fixation, stability, and also on surgeon preference. Activity should be restricted to avoid excessive implant stress.[41] After the immobilization period, initiate hand therapy to regain motion and strength. Serial X-rays and exams should be obtained to assess for any implant loosening or wrist instability. Radiolucency around both the radial and carpal components can be seen; however, alone does not necessarily indicate implant loosening, as stable lucencies of 1 to 2 mm are frequently noted around the articulating platforms.[43] If there is implant migration compared with bony landmarks on serial imaging, this is highly correlated with loosening and foretells the subsequent development of pain.[43]

Outcomes

The natural history of progressive lunate collapse and perilunate arthritis is understood; however, the time course and severity of symptoms can be unpredictable.[44] This has led to a variety of surgical procedures that are difficult to compare as most studies have small case numbers with variable follow-up periods and outcome measures. Currently no specific treatment has been proven in the literature to be superior to another.[45] Lichtman proposed an algorithm for treatment of Kienbock's incorporating various classification systems to help physicians better counsel patients and guide treatment decisions.[16]

Denervation

Schweizer and colleagues reported DASH scores in 70 patients who underwent isolated complete wrist denervation for chronic degenerative wrist pathology, 11 of which had Kienbock's disease. They reported a mean DASH of 26 at over 9 years from surgery for all patients and 24.9 for those with Kienbock's. Forty-eight of 70 reported sustained improvement and would undergo surgery again. Nine patients had an unsatisfactory result requiring additional procedures.[46] Another study reported isolated wrist denervation in 49 patients, 13 of which had Kienbock's disease. Thirty-nine reported improvement in their pain scores and grip strength despite the radiological deterioration in 34 patients after 6 years.[20]

Weinstein and Berger reported outcomes of isolated partial wrist denervation of AIN and PIN neurectomies in 19 patients with an average follow-up of 2.5 years. Eight percent reported decreased pain, 45% normal or increased grip, and 73% returned to work. Three patients required additional procedures for pain relief, including two fusions and one radial styloidectomy. The authors found failures were more common in the first postoperative year.[47]

Proximal row carpectomy

DiDonna et al. performed of series of PRCs in 22 patients, 7 of whom had advanced Kienbock's disease. Patients over 35 years of age maintained satisfactory ROM, grip strength, and pain relief and were overall satisfied with their result. There were four failures that went on to require arthrodesis, all in patients 35 year old or younger, and two of which had Kienbock's disease. They caution performing a PRC in patients under 35 year old given the high rate of radiographic radiocapitate joint degeneration found in long-term follow-up although radiographic findings did not necessarily correlate with outcomes.[25] De

Smet also reported satisfactory outcomes after performing PRC in 21 patients with advanced Kienbock's with an average follow-up of 67 months and no failures.[48] Another study of 12 PRCs in Stage IV Kienbock's with an average of 2-year follow-up reported one failure requiring arthrodesis 3 years after the index surgery.[49]

Croog and colleagues treated 21 wrists with either Stage IIIA, IIIB, and IV Kienbock's with an average follow-up of 10 years. Both average ROM and grip strength were improved; however, three patients went on to require arthrodesis at a mean of 23 months, and two of these three had Stage IV Kienbock's at the time of index surgery. They concluded that while PRC is reliable, higher demand younger patients and those with Stage IV Kienbock's should be advised they may be at high risk for early symptomatic radiocapitate degeneration and need for additional procedures.

Limited intercarpal fusion

STT or SC arthrodesis are commonly described procedures performed in the treatment of advanced Kienbock' disease with satisfactory outcomes. Watson and colleagues reported results of 28 patients treated with STT fusion followed for an average of 51 months and found 78% of patients had good to excellent pain relief and overall improved grip strength and motion.[30] Van den Dungen and colleagues treated patients with either STT arthrodesis or conservative care with a mean follow-up of 13 years. The STT group reported progressive pain, decreased motion, and longer rehabilitation time.[50] Iorio and colleagues performed SC or STT fusion in 12 patients with an average follow-up of 13.1 months and reported significant improvement in postoperative pain scores and bony fusion was obtained in all cases. When compared with case series of patients undergoing PRC, they found average postoperative range of motion after intercarpal fusion to produce similar results.[29] Two of their patients developed CRPS within 100 days of follow-up requiring extensive therapy and desensitization, and one patient required a dorsal capsulotomy for wrist stiffness.[29] Nonunion rates after limited intercarpal fusion are variable, with one metanalysis reporting a nonunion rate of 14%.[51]

When comparing the results of 20 patients who underwent some form of limited intercarpal fusion (n = 13) versus PRC (n = 7), Nakamura and colleagues found no statistical difference in pain, grip strength, or range of motion.[52] This study was limited by the variety of surgical procedures performed as well as variability in disease severity.[52] Tambe and colleagues compared total versus partial wrist intercarpal arthrodesis in patients with either Stage IIIB or IV Kienbock disease.

They found no statistically significant differences in DASH, ROM, or grip strength between the groups; however, four of the partial fusions developed a nonunion requiring revision surgery.[36]

Total wrist arthrodesis

Pain relief after total wrist arthrodesis varies significantly in the literature. De Smet and colleagues reported of 37 wrist fusions, 20 had no pain at rest; however, only six patients remained pain free during activity.[53] Sagerman and colleagues reported outcomes after arthrodesis with a minimum follow-up of 4 years, reporting 17 of 18 patients were satisfied.[54] Weiss and colleagues found that patients who undergo total wrist fusion encounter the most difficulty when in confined spaces and significant wrist flexion is required or when forceful gripping with significant forearm rotation is needed.[55]

Saurbier and colleagues reported outcomes in 60 patients who underwent total wrist arthrodesis for post-traumatic arthritis or Kienbock's disease, with an average follow-up of 37 months. 70% of patients had complete pain relief at rest, whereas 40% were pain free during work. VAS scores were reduced to 55% of preoperative values. Although 80% of patients reported a reduction in their quality of life, 80% also reported they would undergo surgery again.[56]

Complications after total wrist arthrodesis can include wound dehiscence, infection, extensor tendon adhesions, and plate irritation, which can prompt plate removal. Hastings and colleagues compared arthrodesis using plate fixation versus a variety of other methods including intramedullary fixation. Nonunion rate was 2% with plate fixation, versus 18% with other techniques. Complication rate was 51% in plate fixation, versus 79% with alternative fusion techniques.[55] Almost 60% of complications in patients receiving plate fixation required operative treatment, whereas only 21% of alternative technique complications returned to the operating room.[57] Zachary and colleagues reported a 100% union rate after dorsal plate fixation and iliac crest bone grafting but reported 82 complications in 50 of 73 patients. Eighty percent of complications resolved spontaneously or with nonoperative management, whereas 19 required surgery, most commonly for plate removal either due to loosening or irritation.[58]

Wagner and colleagues reported long-term outcomes after bilateral total wrist arthrodesis in 13 patients with an average follow-up of 14 years. Although 93% of patients were satisfied, 7 of 13 required subsequent surgery including five revision arthrodesis and two plate removals. Primary functional limitations included turning a door knob or opening a tight jar lid.[59]

Wrist arthroplasty

Long-term outcomes after TWA are limited for newer generation implants. Cavaliere and colleagues reported better pain relief and less complications in arthrodesis compared with arthroplasty; However, with newer generations, these comparisons have become difficult given limited long-term data.[60] A recent study compared four of the fourth-generation implants and found that all surgeries improved pain and performance. The 5-year survival for the two top performing implants was 90% to 97%, an improvement from prior generations.[61]

Herzberg and colleagues reported outcomes of 215 TWA, 129 in rheumatoid arthritis, and 86 in nonrheumatoid patients, with a survival rate of 96% and 92%, respectively. Each group had improvement in QuickDASH and visual analog pain scores without any statistically significant differences.[62] Weiss and colleagues reported satisfactory pain scores, improved motion, and good to excellent outcomes in 57% of patients with an average follow-up of 27 months in 19 patients using newer generation implants.[41]

Nydick and colleagues compared clinical outcomes after wrist arthrodesis versus TWA in treating pancarpal posttraumatic arthritis. There was no significant difference in DASH or VAS scores; however, specific questions from the PRWE showed statistically significant differences in favor of TWA.[63] A meta-analysis of third-generation arthroplasties found a 21% rate of major complications after TWA versus 13% for arthrodesis.[60] A recent database study found complications to be less frequent, reporting only 10% in TWA versus 7% for arthrodesis.[64]

Carpal component loosening and resultant pain have continued to decrease with new implant designs, and some suggest this may be attributed to the uncemented technique.[41] Intraoperative fractures and deep infections occur in approximately 2% and 1.4% of cases, respectively.[65,66] Although patients undergoing arthrodesis for unsalvageable TWA failure have been shown to have inferior union rates compared with primary fusion, satisfactory results have been reported augmenting the fusion mass with autograft or allograft.[67] Adams and colleagues performed wrist arthrodesis after failed TWA using a shaped femoral head allograft with dorsal plate fixation, resulting in 95% of patients going on to union.[42]

SUMMARY

Kienbock's disease can result in lunate collapse, carpal instability, and eventually perilunate arthritis. There are a variety of wrist salvage procedures described to treat the unreconstructable wrist, and PRC and total wrist arthrodesis are the most commonly described. If considering a motion sparing procedure, PRC, can be performed, however, should be used with caution in younger more active patients who may have accelerated degeneration of the radiocapitate articulation. TWA, although mostly described in treating inflammatory arthritis in the elderly, low-demand populations have become an increasingly popular option with promising results from newer implants. Regardless of the treatment, all patients should be counseled on the expected postoperative limitations both acutely and long term. There remains a need for more dedicated randomized controlled trials comparing these different treatments for advanced Kienbock's disease to help better guide decision making and improve outcomes.

CLINICS CARE POINTS

- Wrist denervation is a motion sparing option for pain relief that can be performed in conjunction with other procedures or in isolation

- PRC is contraindicated in patients with significant cartilage wear of the head of the capitate

- Patients under the age of 35 years who undergo PRC should be counseled; they may be at high risk for revision surgical intervention for progressive symptomatic radiocapitate degeneration

- Performing uncemented versus cemented TWA may allow for easier conversion to total wrist arthrodesis

- TWA should primarily be considered for low demand elderly patients despite the advancement in implant designs

- In cases of post-traumatic or degenerative wrist arthritis, total wrist fusion is a reliable motion sacrificing surgery in which patients achieve a stable wrist with varying degrees of pain relief

- Radiolucencies around radial and carpal components alone do not necessarily indicate loosening after TWA. If implant migration relative to bony landmarks is present on serial imaging, patients are at high risk for loosening and the development of pain

DISCLOSURE

The authors have nothing to disclose.

REFERENCES

1. Cross D, Matullo KS. Kienböck disease. Orthop Clin North Am 2014;45(1):141–52.
2. Gelberman RH, Bauman TD, Menon J, et al. The vascularity of the lunate bone and Kienböck's disease. J Hand Surg Am 1980;5(3):272–8.
3. Allan CH, Joshi A, Lichtman DM. Kienbock's disease: diagnosis and treatment. J Am Acad Orthop Surg 2001;9(2):128–36.
4. Lee ML. The intraosseus arterial pattern of the carpal lunate bone and its relation to avascular necrosis. Acta Orthop Scand 1963;33:43–55.
5. Schiltenwolf M, Martini AK, Mau HC, et al. Further investigations of the intraosseous pressure characteristics in necrotic lunates (Kienb ck's disease). J Hand Surg Am 1996;21(5):754–8.
6. D'Hoore K, De Smet L, Verellen K, et al. Negative ulnar variance is not a risk factor for Kienböck's disease. J Hand Surg Am 1994;19(2):229–31.
7. Divebliss B, Baratz M. Kienbo ck disease. J Am Soc Surg Hand 2001;1:61–72.
8. Takami H, Takahashi S, Ando M, et al. Open reduction of chronic lunate and perilunate dislocations. Arch Orthop Trauma Surg 1996;115:104–7.
9. Ansari MT, Chouhan D, Gupta V, et al. Kienböck's disease: Where do we stand? J Clin Orthop Trauma 2020;11(4):606–13.
10. Mok C, CS L, PW C. Bilateral Kienbock's Disease in SLE. Scand J Rheumatol 1997;26(6):485–7.
11. Matsumoto AK, Moore R, Alli P, et al. Three cases of osteonecrosis of the lunate bone of the wrist in scleroderma. Clin Exp Rheumatol 1999;17:730–2.
12. Ichinose H, Nakamura R, Nakao E, et al. Wrist swelling in Kienböck's disease. J Wrist Surg 2018;7(5):389–93.
13. Lichtman DM, Mack GR, MacDonald RI, et al. Kienböck's disease: the role of silicone replacement arthroplasty. J Bone Joint Surg Am 1977;59:899–908.
14. Kienboeck R. Concerning traumatic malacia of the lunate and its consequences: Degeneration and compression fractures. Clin Orthop Relat Res 1980;149:4–8.
15. Goldfarb CA, Hsu J, Gelberman RH, et al. The Lichtman classification for Kienbock's disease: an assessment of reliability. J Hand Surg 2003;28A:74–80.
16. Lichtman D, Pientka W, Bain G. Addendum: Kienböck Disease: a new algorithm for the 21st century. J Wrist Surg 2017;06(01):e1–2.
17. Lichtman DM, Pientka WF, Bain GI. Kienböck disease: moving forward. J Hand Surg Am 2016;41(5):630–8.
18. Lutsky K, Beredjiklian PK. Kienböck disease. J Hand Surg Am 2012;37(9):1942–52.
19. Wilhelm A. Denervation of the wrist. Tech Hand Up Extrem Surg 2001;5(1):14–30.
20. Braga-Silva J, Roman JA, Padoin AV. Wrist denervation for painful conditions of the wrist. J Hand Surg 2011;36A:961–6.
21. Linscheid RL. Kienböck's disease. Instr Course Lect 1992;41:45–53.
22. Salomon GD, Eaton RG. Proximal row carpectomy with partial capitate resection. J Hand Surg Am 1996;21(1):2–8.
23. Ilyas AM. Proximal row carpectomy with a dorsal capsule interposition flap. Tech Hand Up Extrem Surg 2010;14(3):136–40.
24. Wall LB, Stern PJ. Proximal row carpectomy. Hand Clin 2013;29(1):69–78.
25. DiDonna ML, Kiefhaber TR, Stern PJ. Proximal row carpectomy: study with a minimum of ten years of follow-up. J Bone Joint Surg 2004;86A:2359–65.
26. Stern PJ, Agabegi SS, Kiefhaber TR, et al. Proximal row carpectomy. J Bone Joint Surg 2005;87A:166–74.
27. Berger RA. A method of defining palpable landmarks for the ligament-splitting dorsal wrist capsulotomy. J Hand Surg Am 2007;32(8):1291–5.
28. Iwasaki N, Genda E, Barrance PJ, et al. Biomechical analysis of limited intercarpal 201 fusion for the treatment of Kienböck's disease: a three-dimensional theoretical study. J Orthop Res 1998;16(2):256–63.
29. Iorio ML, Kennedy CD, Huang JI. Limited intercarpal fusion as a salvage procedure for advanced Kienbock disease. Hand 2015;10(3):472–6.
30. Watson HK, Monacelli DM, Milford RS, et al. Treatment of Kienbo ck's disease with scaphotrazio-trapezoid arthrodesis. J Hand Surg Am 1996;21:9–15.
31. Minamikawa Y, Peimer CA, Yamaguchi T, et al. Ideal scaphoid angle for intercarpal arthrodesis. J Hand Surg Am 1992;17:370–5.
32. Hayden RJ, Jebson PJL. Wrist arthrodesis. Hand Clin 2005;21(4):631–40.
33. Rayan GM, Brentlinger A, Purnell D, et al. Functional assessment of bilateral wrist arthrodeses. J Hand Surg Am 1987;12:1020–4.
34. Brumfield RH, Champoux JA. A biomechanical study of normal functional wrist motion. Clin Orthop Relat Res 1984;187:23–5.
35. Clayton ML, Ferlic DC. Arthrodesis of the arthritic wrist. Clin Orthop 1984;187:89–93.
36. Tambe AD, Trail IA, Stanley JK. Wrist fusion versus limited carpal fusion in advanced Kienbock's disease. Int Orthop 2005;29(6):355–8.
37. Luboshitz S, Burstein G, Engel J. Wrist arthrodesis : modified Gill ' S technique. J Hand Surg Br 2002;27(6):568–72.
38. Jebson PJ, Adams BD. Wrist arthrodesis: review of current technique. J Am Acad Orthop Surg 2001;9(1):53–60.
39. Wysocki RW, Cohen MS. Complications of limited and total wrist arthrodesis. Hand Clin 2010;26(2):221–8.
40. Lin HH, Stern PJ. Salvage" procedures in the treatment of Kienbock's disease. Proximal row

carpectomy and total wrist arthrodesis. Hand Clin 1993;9:521–6.

41. Weiss AP, Kamal RN, Shultz P. Total wrist arthroplasty. J Am Acad Orthop Surg 2013;21(3):140e148.

42. Adams BD, Kleinhenz BP, Guan JJ. Wrist arthrodesis for failed total wrist arthroplasty. J Hand Surg Am 2016;41(6):673e679.

43. Halim A, Weiss APC. Total wrist arthroplasty. J Hand Surg Am 2017;42(3):198–209.

44. Croog AS, Stern PJ. Proximal row carpectomy for advanced Kienbock's Disease: average 10-year follow-up. J Hand Surg Am 2008;33(7):1122–30.

45. Innes L, Strauch RJ. Systematic review of the treatment of Kienbock's disease in its early and late stages. J Hand Surg 2010;35A:713–7. e711–e714.

46. Schweizer A, von Kanel O, Kammer E, et al. Long-term follow-up evaluation of denervation of the wrist. J Hand Surg 2006;31A:559–64.

47. Weinstein LP, Berger RA. Analgesic benefit, functional outcome, and patient satisfaction after partial wrist denervation. J Hand Surg Am 2002;27(5):833–9.

48. De Smet L, Robijns P, Degreef I. Proximal row carpectomy in advanced Kienbock's disease. J Hand Surg 2005;30B:585–7.

49. El-Mowafi H, El-Hadidi M, El-Karef E. Proximal row carpectomy: a motion-preserving procedure in the treatment of advanced Kienbock's disease. Acta Orthop Belg 2006;72:530–4.

50. Van den Dungen S, Dury M, Foucher G, et al. Conservative treatment versus scaphotrapeziotrapezoid arthrodesis for Kienbo ck's disease. a retrospective study. Chir Main 2006;25:141–5.

51. Larsen CF, Jacoby RA, McCabe SJ. Nonunion rates of limited carpal arthrodesis: a meta-analysis of the literature. J Hand Surg Am 1997;22:66–73.

52. Nakamura R, Horii E, Watanabe K. Proximal row carpectomy versus limited wrist arthrodesis for advanced Kienbo ck's disease. J Hand Surg Br 1998;23:741–5.

53. De Smet L, Truyen J. Arthrodesis of the wrist for osteoarthritis: outcome with a minimum follow-up of 4 years. J Hand Surg Br 2003;28(6):575–7.

54. Sagerman SD, Palmer AK. Wrist arthrodesis using a dynamic compression plate. J Hand Surg Br 1996;21(4):437–41.

55. Weiss APC, Wiedeman G, Quenzer D, et al. Upper extremity function after wrist arthrodesis. J Hand Surg Am 1995;20(5):813–7.

56. Sauerbier M, Kluge S, Bickert B, et al. Subjective and objective outcomes after total wrist arthrodesis in patients with radiocarpal arthrosis or Kienböck's disease. Chir Main 2000;19(4):223–31.

57. Hastings H II, Weiss APC, Quenzer D, et al. Arthrodesis of the wrist for post-traumatic disorders. J Bone Joint Surg Am 1996;78:897–902.

58. Zachary SV, Stern PJ. Complications following AO/ASIF wrist arthrodesis. J Hand Surg Am 1995;20(2):339–44.

59. Wagner ER, Elhassan BT, Kakar S. Long-term functional outcomes after bilateral total wrist arthrodesis. J Hand Surg Am 2015;40(2):224–228 e1.

60. Cavaliere CM, Chung KC. A systematic review of total wrist arthroplasty compared with total wrist arthrodesis for rheumatoid arthritis. Plast Reconstr Surg 2008;122(3):813e825.

61. Sagerfors M, Gupta A, Brus O, et al. Patient related functional outcome after total wrist arthroplasty: a single center study of 206 cases. Hand Surg 2015;20(1):81e87.

62. Herzberg G, Boeckstyns M, Sorensen AI, et al. Remotion" total wrist arthroplasty: preliminary results of a prospective international multicenter study of 215 cases. J Wrist Surg 2012;1(1):17e22.

63. Nydick JA, Watt JF, Garcia MJ, et al. Clinical outcomes of arthrodesis and arthroplasty for the treatment of posttraumatic wrist arthritis. J Hand Surg Am 2013;38(5):899e903.

64. Melamed E, Marascalchi B, Hinds RM, et al. Trends in the utilization of total wrist arthroplasty versus wrist fusion for treatment of advanced wrist arthritis. J Wrist Surg 2016;5(3):211e216.

65. Wagner ER, Mehrotra K, Rizzo M. Intraoperative and postoperative fractures in total wrist arthroplasty: risk factors and long-term outcomes. J Hand Surg 2015;40(9S):e51ee52.

66. Boeckstyns ME. Wrist arthroplasty—a systematic review. Dan Med J 2014;61(5):A4834.

67. Rizzo M, Ackerman DB, Rodrigues RL, et al. Wrist arthrodesis as a salvage procedure for failed implant arthroplasty. J Hand Surg Eur Vol 2011;36(1):29–33.

Arthroscopic Management of Kienböck Disease

Eric R. Wagner, MD, Alexander R. Graf, MD*

KEYWORDS

- Lunate avascular necrosis • Kienböck disease • Wrist arthroscopy • Carpal collapse
- Carpal instability • Wrist arthritis

KEY POINTS

- Wrist arthroscopy is a useful diagnostic and treatment tool for patients with Kienböck disease of all stages.
- Arthroscopic treatment for early Kienböck disease requires intact lunate articular surfaces and aims to improve pain and motion while limiting disease progression.
- Arthroscopic treatment for advanced Kienböck disease is technically demanding but potentially facilitates faster patient recovery and less pain due to minimal capsular disruption and scarring.

INTRODUCTION

The development of smaller arthroscopes and instrumentation to accommodate the wrist in the 1980s revolutionized the understanding and treatment of a myriad of hand and wrist disorders.[1] For the first time, the radiocarpal and midcarpal articulations as well as surrounding ligaments could be visualized arthroscopically using a short-barrel 50- to 60-mm scope with an outside diameter of 2 to 3 mm at an angle of 25° to 30°. In addition, wrist arthroscopy procedures allowed for less surgical dissection, decreased postoperative pain, a shorter recovery time, and an earlier return to work for patients.[1] However, wrist arthroscopy was not used in the management of Kienböck disease until Menth-Chiari used it to assess the articular surfaces, debride the necrotic lunate and degenerative ligaments, and perform a limited synovectomy in 1999.[2] In their study of 7 patients, all were either Lichtman grade IIIA or IIIB, and all experienced relief of their painful mechanical symptoms.

Since that time, the diagnostic and therapeutic applications of wrist arthroscopy in the management of Kienböck disease have significantly increased.[3] Through direct visualization and inspection of the chondral surface, a better understanding of the pathoanatomy of Kienböck disease enables surgeons to be more precise when making the ultimate treatment decision, which has potentially improved the ultimate treatment algorithm.[4]

DIAGNOSTIC APPROACH

The utility of wrist arthroscopy in the diagnosis and staging of Kienböck disease stems from its ability to directly assess the integrity of the chondral surfaces upon and surrounding the lunate, which are often misunderstood based on radiographic assessment and clinical findings.[5,6] This is performed using standard wrist arthroscopic techniques and the 3-4, 6R, and both midcarpal portals (**Fig. 1**).[3] The patient is positioned supine on the operating room table under general anesthesia with the extremity extended on an arm table. A brachial tourniquet is applied but seldom needed unless bleeding obstructs visualization. A general assessment of the radiocarpal and midcarpal joints is first performed, noting the presence or absence of synovitis or loose bodies. Synovitis

Disclosure: The authors have nothing to disclose.
Emory University, Department of Orthopedic Surgery, Division of Upper Extremity Surgery, Emory Orthopaedics & Spine Center, 21 Ortho Lane, Atlanta, GA 30329, USA
* Corresponding author:
E-mail address: Alexander.reed.graf@emory.edu

Hand Clin 38 (2022) 461–468
https://doi.org/10.1016/j.hcl.2022.03.008

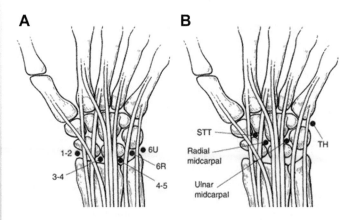

Fig. 1. Standard wrist arthroscopic portals. R, radial; STT, scaphotrapeziotrapezoid; U, ulnar. (*Adapted from* Gupta R, Bozentka DJ, Osterman AL. Wrist arthroscopy: principles and clinical applications. J Am Acad Orthop Surg. 2001;9(3):200-209. doi:10.5435/00124635-200105000-00006; with permission)

is often present in patients with Kienböck disease and has previously been correlated with the degree of articular damage around the lunate and surrounding articulations.[6] First, the 3-4 portal is used for visualization and the 6R portal is used as the working portal, allowing the surgeon to assess the proximal lunate, lunate fossa, radioscaphoid (RS) articulation, triangular fibrocartilage complex (TFCC), and proximal synovium. Next, the midcarpal arthroscopy is performed using the midcarpal ulnar (MCU) portal for visualization and the midcarpal radial (MCR) portal for instruments. The distal lunate and proximal capitate are inspected, as well as the rest of the midcarpus. The lunate surfaces are palpated with a probe and the presence of softening, "floating" (unsupported) articular surface, or gross degenerative changes are noted. Normal articular cartilage should appear white, firm, and smooth (**Fig. 2**). Degenerative articular changes in Kienböck disease include chondral fibrillation, sclerosis, fissuring, localized or extensive loss, a floating articular surface, or even fracture in advanced disease (**Fig. 3**).[6]

Differentiating normal from degenerative cartilage changes during wrist arthroscopy helps define "functional" from "nonfunctional" articulations.[3] This also serves as the foundation for the Bain and Begg classification system, which defines the patient's specific pathoanatomy and informs treatment selection (**Fig. 4**).[6] According to their classification system, pathologic changes generally start at the convex proximal lunate surface, and then progress to the adjacent lunate fossa of the radius, and then the remainder of the central column of the wrist.[3] The incidence of chondral lesions is associated with increased age and duration of disease.[7] The stage corresponds with number of "nonfunctional" articulations, which must be either excised, bypassed, or fused for successful treatment.[3]

In addition to assessment of chondral changes, wrist arthroscopy in the setting of Kienböck disease also affords the ability to directly assess and address additional intracarpal pathology. In a study of 32 wrists with Kienböck disease, Watanabe demonstrated that tears of the scapholunate (SL) and/or lunotriquetral (LT) interosseous ligaments were present 50% of the time, with incidence being directly correlated with disease stage.[8] In addition, TFCC tears were also common and associated with age over 30 years (44% of patients) and positive ulnar variance (60% of patients).

ARTHROSCOPIC TREATMENT OF EARLY DISEASE

The pathologic changes in Kienböck disease are thought to occur in 3 phases. The early vascular phase is characterized by ischemia, necrosis, and revascularization. This is followed by an intermediate osseous phase, characterized by sclerosis, subchondral collapse, coronal fracture, and remodeling.[6] The final phase, or late chondral phase, is characterized by subchondral bone collapse, chondral degeneration, and adjacent carpal chondral degeneration.

In patients with early disease, in which diagnostic arthroscopy reveals intact functional articulations, treatment is focused on limiting progression of disease. In patients who have failed conservative treatment, arthroscopic treatment options include debridement with synovectomy, forage, and arthroscopic-assisted bone grafting, as well as arthroscopic intercarpal fusions.

Forage

In early disease when functional articulations are spared, synovectomy is often performed at the time of arthroscopic forage. The arthroscopic forage (drilling) procedure is borne out of the idea

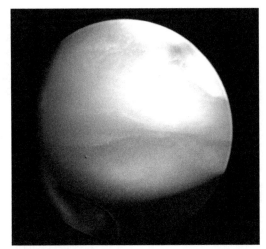

Fig. 2. Functional proximal lunate chondral surface visualized adjacent to shaver. Chondral surface is white, firm, and smooth.

that venous congestion contributes to increased intraosseous pressure and contributes to early avascular necrosis (AVN).[9] Therefore, just as core decompression has been shown to be effective in femoral and humeral head AVN, Bain and colleagues[9] have described an arthroscopic lunate core decompression for patients with early disease (Bain and Begg stage 0), neutral or positive ulnar variance, and no lunate collapse on plain radiographs. To perform this procedure, the 3-4 and 6R portals are used to debride synovitis with an arthroscopic shaver and assess the lunate and adjacent articulations. Then, switching the scope to the 6R portal, and the 3-4 portal is used to drill

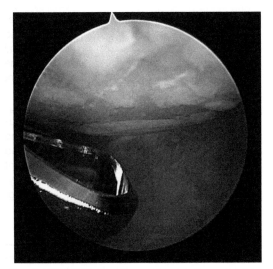

Fig. 3. Chondral fissuring and sclerosis present on nonfunctional proximal lunate articulation as viewed through 3-4 portal.

the dorsal aspect of the lunate through a cannula (**Fig. 5**). In their series of 2 patients with long-term follow-up, both patients had significant improvement in pain and range of motion at 6-year follow-up. However, despite their excellent clinical results, radiographs showed progression to lunate collapse in one of the patients.[9]

More recently, capitate forage has been introduced as an idea to improve lunate vascularity, similar to distal radius core decompression.[10] Although the initial technique proposed is a percutaneous one with fluoroscopic guidance, this is now performed using wrist arthroscopy, viewing through the MCU portal and drilling via the MCR portal or an accessory distal portal. Early results in 9 patients showed maintained wrist motion, improvement in pain, and moderate patient satisfaction. Furthermore, given its low complication profile compared with capitate- and distal radius-based osteotomies, it warrants consideration in the early Kienböck disease treatment algorithm.

Bone Grafting

For patients with intact functional articulations but evidence of lunate osteonecrosis or hypovascularity without collapse, arthroscopic bone grafting allows for lunate decompression, as well as debridement and application of bone-forming elements. The technique involves diagnostic arthroscopy used first to confirm functional articulations utilizing 3-4 and 6R portals. In the absence of a lunate chondral lesion, the proximal insertion of the LT ligament is opened using a 3 mm burr to debride nonviable lunate bone. Once this has been completed, a trocar is inserted in the defect and bone graft is packed using a plunger or trocar. In Pegoli's technique, cancellous graft is harvested from volar radius and inserted through a trocar placed through 3-4 portal into lunate cavity while viewing through the 6R portal (**Fig. 6**).[11] In their study of 3 patients with Lichtman stage I disease with an average 13.5-month follow-up, all patients had improved pain and wrist function, as well as lunate vascularity on postoperative MRI.[11]

More recently, Rajfer and colleagues[12] have introduced the novel application of bone morphogenic protein (BMP)-2 on collagen carrier scaffold for treatment of arthroscopically staged IIIA/B patients with ulnar-neutral or ulnar-positive variance. In their technique, the BMP-2 is inserted through a window created in lunate with a burr near the LT ligament insertion, and then packed with an autologous bone graft from the distal radius or iliac crest. Although early results are promising, there remains a paucity of midterm and long-term results.

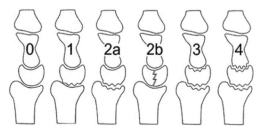

Fig. 4. Arthroscopic classification of avascular necrosis of the lunate. (*Adapted from* Bain GI, Begg M. Arthroscopic assessment and classification of Kienbock's disease. Tech Hand Up Extrem Surg. 2006;10(1):8-13. doi:10.1097/00130911-200603000-00003; with permission)

ARTHROSCOPIC TREATMENT OF ADVANCED DISEASE

Arthroscopic treatment of advanced disease depends on the number of remaining functional articulations present. With proximal lunate and/or distal radius lunate facet involvement (Bain and Begg stage 1 and 2), arthroscopic (or open) radioscapholunate (RSL) fusion as well as proximal row carpectomy (PRC) are reliable and reproducible.[6] When additional functional articulations are involved (stages 3 and 4), arthroscopic (or open) lunate excision with scaphocapitate fusion are options as alternatives to traditional open techniques, such as total wrist fusion or wrist arthroplasty.[13] Arthroscopic debridement to improve pain and mechanical symptoms has also been described with moderate results, but less morbidity.[14]

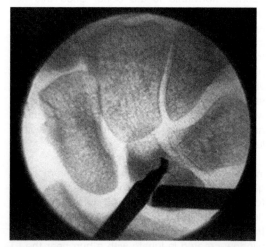

Fig. 5. Arthroscopic forage procedure using 2 mm drill placed through 3-4 portal with fluoroscopic guidance. (*From* Bain GI, Durrant A. An articular-based approach to Kienbock avascular necrosis of the lunate. Tech Hand Up Extrem Surg. 2011;15(1):41-47. doi:10.1097/BTH.0b013e31820e82e8; with permission)

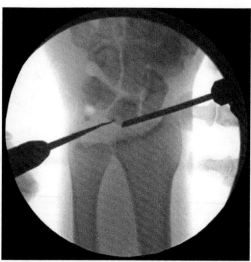

Fig. 6. Arthroscopic bone grafting for early Kienböck disease. While viewing through the 3-4 portal, a 4 mm burr is inserted through 6R portal to create hole for graft near the lunate insertion of the LT ligament. Graft is harvested and packed through 3 mm cannula to the edge of cortical bone. (*From* Pegoli L, Ghezzi A, Cavalli E, Luchetti R, Pajardi G. Arthroscopic assisted bone grafting for early stages of Kienböck's disease. Hand Surg Int J Devoted Hand Up Limb Surg Relat Res J Asia-Pac Fed Soc Surg Hand. 2011;16(2):127-131. doi:10.1142/S0218810411005436; with permission)

RSL Fusion

To consider an RSL fusion, it is required to have a functional lunocapitate joint. According to Bain, the procedure is performed using 1-2, 3-4, and 4-5 portals.[3] With the scope in the 4–5 portal, and the burr in the 1–2 and 3–4 portals, the radial styloid and scaphoid fossa, as well as overhanging proximal scaphoid and lunate surfaces, are debrided to the healthy subchondral bone as joint preparation for fusion.[3] Bone graft is harvested and delivered via the 4.5 mm cannula through the 1–2 and 3–4 portals and compacted tightly into the radiocarpal space given the size mismatch between the radius, scaphoid, and lunate. The wrist is taken out of traction, and guidewires for percutaneous cannulated compression screws are then placed under fluoroscopic guidance across RS and radiolunate (RL) articulations (**Fig. 7**).[14] The RL pin is introduced 1 cm proximal to the dorsal rim of the radius and aimed at the volar horn of the lunate, to maximize lunate purchase, but to avoid penetration and associated danger to the median nerve. The RS pin is introduced into the radial column toward the proximal scaphoid at 45° on the anteroposterior view. On the lateral view, the pin is aimed along the mid axis of radial styloid and

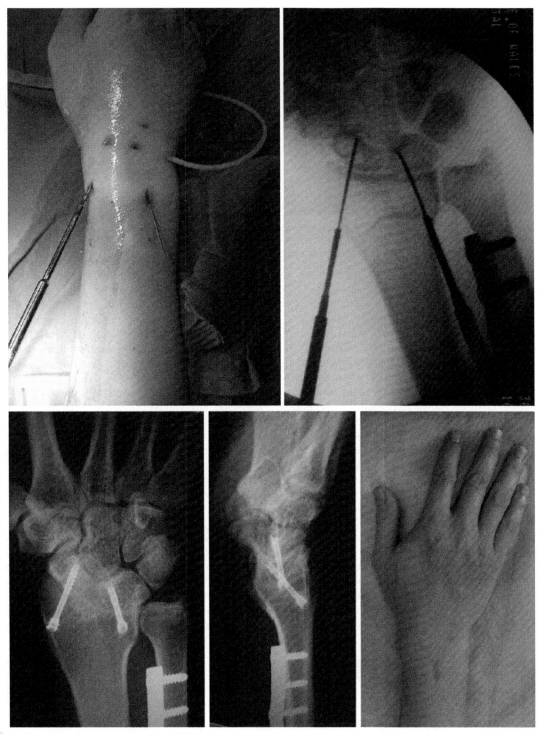

Fig. 7. Arthroscopic technique for RSL fusion (above). Final radiographic and clinical outcome at 39 months (below). (*From* Ho PC. Arthroscopic partial wrist fusion. Tech Hand Up Extrem Surg. 2008;12(4):242-265. doi:10.1097/BTH.0b013e318190244b; with permission)

proximal scaphoid. Furthermore, although Ertem and colleagues[13] reported successful fusion at 7 weeks in 11 patients without the use of bone graft with arthroscopic scaphocapitate fusion, comparative arthroscopic RSL fusion rates using a necrotic lunate are not currently known.

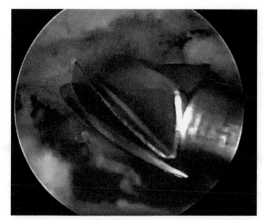

Fig. 8. Arthroscopic view of hooded burr debriding proximal lunate in 3-4 portal while viewing from 6R portal during arthroscopic proximal row carpectomy.

Proximal Row Carpectomy

Arthroscopic PRC requires an intact proximal capitate and lunate facet of the distal radius. It was first described by Culp and colleagues, in 1997, and although technically challenging, can result in potentially improved functional results and an accelerated rehabilitation when compared with the open traditional technique.[15,16] An additional benefit is preserved dorsal capsular innervation and integrity, which is thought to improve wrist proprioception and radiocapitate stability.[17]

The technique involves routine radiocarpal and midcarpal arthroscopy carried out using the 3-4, 6R, MCR, and MCU portals. The procedure is started by using the 6R viewing portal and 3-4 working portal, using first a 2.9 mm burr and then a 4.0 mm hooded burr to start to remove the proximal scaphoid and lunate (**Fig. 8**). The view and working portals are then switched, and then the proximal triquetrum is burred. Next, using the MCU viewing portal and MCR working portal, the distal scaphoid, lunate, and triquetrum are excised. This is started by using a small shaver

or burr to begin the carpectomy at the medial corner of the scaphoid at the midcarpal SL joint, with care to preserve the articular cartilage of the proximal capitate. Then, the portal is enlarged and a 4 mm hooded bur is introduced into the midcarpal joint. The scaphoid is then removed from ulnar to radial and distal to proximal. The viewing and working portals are switched. The scaphotrapeziotrapezoid (STT) portal is used to facilitate removal of the distal pole of the scaphoid while viewing in the MCR portal. After scaphoid excision, the arthroscope is placed in the STT or MCR portal. The burr is placed in an enlarged MCR or MCU portal, and then the lunate (distal to proximal) and triquetrum (distal to proximal) are sequentially removed (**Fig. 9**).[15] An accessory volar central portal can also be used to expedite bone excision and improve dorsal carpus visualization but is not routinely performed.[17] Arthroscopic radial styloidectomy can also be performed to improve radial deviation with the burr in the 1-2 portal and the arthroscope in the 3-4 portal. Patients are immobilized in soft dressing postoperatively and encouraged to being immediate wrist range of motion with a removable splint for comfort.

In a series of 16 patients with an average 2-year follow-up, patients had significant improvement in pain and function, with an average wrist flexion-extension arc of 80% and grip strength of 81% on the contralateral side.[15] In addition, the learning curve in the series ranged from surgical times of 90 to 120 minutes early in the series, to 30 to 40 minutes in the latter cases.

Scaphocapitate Fusion

Scaphocapitate fusion requires a functional RS articulation for motion and aims to offload the lunate to improve pain and prevent disease progression in the earlier stages of Kienböck disease.[3] It is preferred to STT fusion, given its easier access arthroscopically and direct bypass

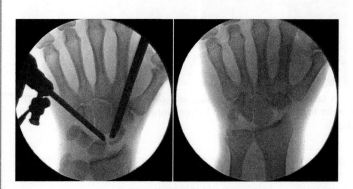

Fig. 9. Arthroscopic proximal row carpectomy. Burr is used to first debride medial scaphoid waist (left), followed by remaining scaphoid, lunate and triquetrum (right). (*From* Weiss ND, Molina RA, Gwin S. Arthroscopic proximal row carpectomy. J Hand Surg. 2011;36(4):577-582. doi:10.1016/j.jhsa.2011.01.009; with permission)

of the diseased articulations. To perform this procedure, MCU, MCR, and STT portals are used. The opposing surfaces of the scaphoid and capitate are debrided down to bleeding subchondral bone, viewing in the MCU and working in the MCR. The radial aspect of the articulation is prepared by viewing through the MCR and working through the STT. Intraoperatively, fluoroscopy is used to maintain normal carpal alignment (SL angle: 30°–57° and capitolunate angle: 0°–15°).[3] Two guide pins are inserted across the scaphocapitate interval percutaneously. The first guide pin is advanced through the 1–2 portal and should enter the scaphoid between the proximal and middle thirds at a 60° angle to the longitudinal axis of the wrist. The second guide pin is inserted at least 5 mm distal and parallel to the first wire, aiming to enter the scaphoid between the middle and distal thirds. Cannulated compressions screws are then drilled, measured, and inserted across the prepared joint to facilitate fusion.[3]

In patients with advanced Kienböck disease with proximal capitate involvement, lunate excision with scaphocapitate fusion offers a minimally invasive and motion-sparing alternative to wrist fusion. In 2016, Ertem reported his series of 11 patients with Bain and Begg stage 3 and 4 Kienböck disease who underwent arthroscopic lunate excision and scaphocapitate fusion without bone graft.[13] In his series, all patients had improvement in pain and function at 6 -month follow-up, there were no complications and fusion occurred after 7 weeks on average. However, given the limited follow-up, long-term outcomes and the effect of surgery on disease progression could not be determined.

Debridement

For patients with advanced disease and nonfunctional articulations, articular debridement with removal of synovitis and loose bodies can help relieve pain and mechanical symptoms. This option is ideally suited for patients who are otherwise not good surgical candidates for open salvage options, such as wrist arthroplasty or total wrist fusion.

The technique uses 1–2, 3–4, and 6R portals alternately used as both working and viewing portals and a 2.4-mm, 30° arthroscope. Debridement of synovial tissue, radiocarpal septa, loose bodies, chondral flaps, and interosseous ligament tears is performed using a combination of shaver and radiofrequency ablation device.[18] Arthrolysis can also be performed to remove adhesions in the radiocarpal joint and release the dorsal and volar radiocarpal ligaments as well as the capsule of the wrist joint from the radial attachments.

Recently, Ayik and colleagues[18] published their results on 15 patients with Lichtman stage III and IV Kienböck disease who underwent arthroscopic debridement and arthrolysis. They found significant improvement in pain, wrist range of motion, and grip strength at an average follow-up of 36 months despite evidence of disease progression on radiographs. They concluded that arthroscopic debridement is a relatively fast, safe, and effective treatment option, which may delay the need for more invasive salvage procedures in the future.

DIRECTIONS FOR FURTHER RESEARCH

Although wrist arthroscopy has recently emerged as a helpful diagnostic and treatment tool for patients with Kienböck disease, comparative studies between arthroscopic and traditional open methods of treatment are lacking. In addition, it is unclear which arthroscopic treatments (if any) alter the natural history of the disease, and how radiographic progression influences the development of clinical symptoms. Future multicenter prospective studies will be required to answer some of these questions to determine the optimal treatment of Kienböck disease moving forward.

SUMMARY

- Radiographic changes in Kienböck disease often do not correlate with arthroscopic and clinical findings
- Wrist arthroscopy enables a more precise diagnosis and can help surgeons select the most appropriate treatment option
- Arthroscopic techniques are an effective treatment option for early and advanced Kienböck disease
- Owing to the less invasive nature of wrist arthroscopic procedures, their utility is likely to increase in the future to promote improved early rehabilitation and function.

CLINICS CARE POINTS

- Patients with Kienböck disease have variable clinical presentations and examination findings
- Radiographs often underestimate the degree of chondral injury

- Wrist arthroscopy is minimally invasive and allows for accurate staging and treatment of Kienböck disease
- Arthroscopic treatment options for Kienböck disease are effective for both early and advanced disease

REFERENCES

1. Gupta R, Bozentka DJ, Osterman AL. Wrist arthroscopy: principles and clinical applications. J Am Acad Orthop Surg 2001;9(3):200–9.
2. Menth-Chiari WA, Poehling GG, Wiesler ER, et al. Arthroscopic debridement for the treatment of Kienbock's disease. Arthroscopy 1999;15(1):12–9.
3. Bain GI, Begg M. Arthroscopic assessment and classification of Kienbock's disease. Tech Hand Up Extrem Surg 2006;10(1):8–13.
4. MacLean SBM, Bain GI. Long-term outcome of surgical treatment for Kienböck Disease using an articular-based classification. J Hand Surg 2021; 46(5):386–95.
5. Pillukat T, Kalb K, van Schoonhoven J, et al. [The value of wrist arthroscopy in Kienböck's disease]. Handchir Mikrochir Plast Chir Organ Deutschsprachigen Arbeitsgemeinschaft Handchir Organ Deutschsprachigen Arbeitsgemeinschaft Mikrochir Peripher Nerven Gefasse Organ V 2010;42(3): 204–11. https://doi.org/10.1055/s-0030-1253407.
6. Bain GI, Durrant A. An articular-based approach to Kienbock avascular necrosis of the lunate. Tech Hand Up Extrem Surg 2011;15(1):41–7.
7. Tatebe M, Hirata H, Shinohara T, et al. Arthroscopic findings of Kienböck's disease. J Orthop Sci 2011; 16(6):745–8.
8. Watanabe K, Nakamura R, Imaeda T. Arthroscopic assessment of Kienböck's disease. Arthrosc J Arthrosc Relat Surg 1995;11(3):257–62.
9. Bain GI, Smith ML, Watts AC. Arthroscopic core decompression of the lunate in early stage Kienbock disease of the lunate. Tech Hand Up Extrem Surg 2011;15(1):66–9.
10. Bekler HI, Erdag Y, Gumustas SA, et al. The proposal and early results of capitate forage as a new treatment method for Kienböck's disease. J Hand Microsurg 2013;5(2):58–62.
11. Pegoli L, Ghezzi A, Cavalli E, et al. Arthroscopic assisted bone grafting for early stages of Kienböck's disease. Hand Surg 2011;16(2):127–31. https://doi.org/10.1142/S0218810411005436.
12. Rajfer RA, Danoff JR, Metzl JA, et al. A novel arthroscopic technique utilizing bone morphogenetic protein in the treatment of Kienböck disease. Tech Hand Up Extrem Surg 2013;17(1):2–6.
13. Ertem K, Görmeli G, Karakaplan M, et al. Arthroscopic limited intercarpal fusion without bone graft in patients with Kienböck's disease. Eklem Hastalik Cerrahisi 2016;27(3):132–7.
14. Ho PC. Arthroscopic partial wrist fusion. Tech Hand Up Extrem Surg 2008;12(4):242–65.
15. Weiss ND, Molina RA, Gwin S. Arthroscopic proximal row carpectomy. J Hand Surg 2011;36(4): 577–82.
16. Culp RW, Lee Osterman A, Talsania JS. Arthroscopic proximal row carpectomy. Tech Hand Up Extrem Surg 1997;1(2):116–9.
17. Ocampos Hernandez M, Corella Montoya F, Del Cerro Gutierrez M, et al. Arthroscopic proximal row carpectomy using the volar central portal. Arthrosc Tech 2017;6(4):e1427–30.
18. Ayik O, Demirel M, Turgut N, et al. Arthroscopic debridement and arthrolysis for the treatment of advanced Kienböck's disease: 18-Month and 5-year postoperative results. J Wrist Surg 2021;10(4): 280–5.

Preiser's Disease—Current Concepts of Etiology and Management

Simon F. Bellringer, MBBS, BSc, FRCS(Tr&Orth)[a],
Simon B.M. MacLean, MBChB, FRCS(Tr&Orth), PGDipCE[b],
Gregory I. Bain, PhD, MBBS, FRACS, FA(Ortho)A[c],*

KEYWORDS

• Preiser's disease • Scaphoid • Avascular necrosis • Osteonecrosis

KEY POINTS

• The term Preiser's disease should be used exclusively to describe idiopathic avascular necrosis of the scaphoid.
• Preiser's disease is rare and the natural history is not fully understood.
• After history and clinical examination, CT (4D), MRI and arthoscopy have an important role in the assessment of the scaphoid, surrounding carpus and any associated carpal instability.
• Management should be based on patient factors as well as the stage of the disease within the scaphoid and the surrounding wrist.

▶ Video content accompanies this article at http://www.hand.theclinics.com.

BACKGROUND

Preiser's disease is defined as 'idiopathic avascular necrosis (AVN) of the scaphoid'. Georg Preiser (1876–1913) was an orthopedic surgeon based in Hamburg. He first published an article in 1910,[1] where he described 24 cases of scaphoid fracture. In five of these cases, he found the radiographs to be different with no evidence of primary fracture and 'rarifying osteitis' akin to AVN and suggested a pathologic process involving ligament rupture, blood vessel rupture, bone weakening, osteoporosis, sclerosis, and ultimately fracture of the scaphoid. In 1911,[2] Preiser related his own findings to those of Kienbock's lunomalacia and Kohler's disease of the navicular.

Kallen and Strackee[3] had contrasting views of the condition. They reviewed Preiser's original work over 100 years later and found pathology suggestive of primary fracture and little compelling evidence of idiopathic AVN in all five cases originally described (**Fig. 1**A, B). Interestingly, they were not the first to have made these observations, with one of Preiser's peers, a Dr Haenish, noting fractures lines present on radiographs; findings that were refuted by Preiser in his second paper.[4] Herbert and Lanzetta[5] also noted that Preiser's cases were all secondary to a history of trauma in 1993 but did not comment on the original images. Therefore, despite contemporaneous and retrospective peer review suggesting a primary traumatic pathology in his original description,

---

[a] Department of Orthopaedic Surgery and Trauma, Flinders Medical Centre, Bedford Park, South Australia, Australia; [b] Department of Orthopaedic Surgery, Tauranga Hospital, Bay of Plenty, New Zealand; [c] Department of Orthopaedic Surgery and Trauma, Flinders Medical Centre, Flinders University, Bedford Park, South Australia, Australia
* Corresponding author. 196 Melbourne Street, North Adelaide, South Australia 5006, Australia.
E-mail address: admin@gregbain.com.au

Hand Clin 38 (2022) 469–477
https://doi.org/10.1016/j.hcl.2022.03.013

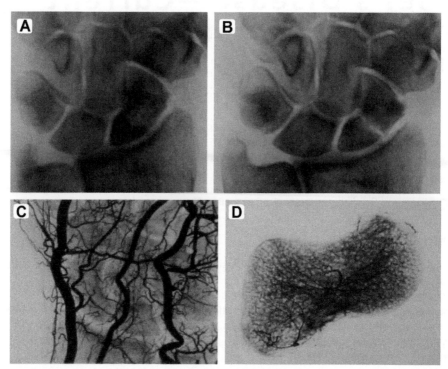

Fig. 1. (*A, B*) Radiographs from the case of a 30-year-old man from Preiser's original paper in 1910: (*A*) Right wrist radiograph was taken at 7 months postinjury demonstrating evidence of primary scaphoid waist fracture with cyst formation. (*B*) Right wrist radiograph taken at 15 months postinjury demonstrating nonunion. (*C, D*) Injection techniques and radiographs to visualize the blood supply to the scaphoid. (*From* Kallen AM, Strackee SD. On the history and definition of Preiser's disease. J Hand Surg Eur Vol. 2014;39(7):770-776. https://doi.org/10.1177/1753193413501099; with permission.)

the term Preiser's disease is still most frequently used to describe 'idiopathic AVN of the scaphoid'.

Perhaps in keeping with its rather chaotic history, Preiser's disease has also been used to describe avascular necrosis of the scaphoid where the cause is reported to be known including that of trauma, systemic disease, smoking, chemotherapy, and steroid use.[6–13]

The authors of the chapter would therefore suggest that the term Preiser's disease be used to describe exclusively idiopathic AVN of the scaphoid.

Incidence

Preiser's disease is exceedingly rare with a recent systematic literature review identifying only 170 cases. It is slightly more common in women (58%) and can occur in a wide range of age groups (9–76 years) with no peak of frequency observed. It occurs in the dominant wrist twice as often as the nondominant wrist.[14]

Clinical Presentation

Presentation tends to be nonspecific, with an insidious onset of dorso-radial-sided wrist pain

(50% of patients) or swelling (19%) over a number of months (mean 31 months) at first presentation.[14] Patients often present at advanced stages of the disease, as symptoms are often misdiagnosed initially as a "wrist sprain". In advanced stages, generalized stiffness predominates, due to degenerative changes in the carpus.

Physical examination may reveal tenderness over the scaphoid and restricted range of movement or function in the affected wrist.[15] There are no specific clinical "special tests" for the disease.

Investigations

Radiographs

Radiographs should be performed in all patients. Standard posteroanterior and lateral radiographs are required to look for evidence of scaphoid sclerosis, fracture, fragmentation, and periscaphoid arthritis changes. These form the basis of Herbert's classification of the disease in **Table 1**.[5]

Magnetic resonance imaging

Magnetic resonance imaging (MRI) provides both diagnostic and prognostic value. Kalainov[16] described 2 types of Preiser's disease based on contrast-enhanced MRI scans performed in their

Table 1
Herbert classification of Preiser's disease based on radiographs

Stage	Radiographic Findings
Stage 1	Normal (positive bone scintigraphy only)
Stage 2	Increased density in the proximal pole. Generalized osteoporosis
Stage 3	Fragmentation of the proximal pole ± pathologic fracture
Stage 4	Carpal collapse ± osteoarthritis

case series of 19 patients. Type 1 involved necrosis/ischemia of the entire scaphoid (**Fig. 2**A), while type 2 involves segmental vascular impairment of the scaphoid (**Fig. 3**A). They found that in type 1 scaphoids, all had a poor outcome regardless of treatment strategy resulting in scaphoid fragmentation and carpal collapse, while those with type 2 scaphoids had a decreased tendency toward fragmentation and had more favorable clinical outcomes in their series.

Schmitt[17] described variations in MRI findings seen in seven patients with Preiser's disease identifying three distinct areas of disease within an affected scaphoid; at the proximal pole of the scaphoid 'zone of osteonecrosis' (with no T1 or T2 signal), in the middle of the scaphoid 'zone of repair' with evidence of hypervascularity (with increased T1 signal), and the distal pole with a 'zone of viable bone marrow' with normal T1 and T2 signals (**Fig. 4**). They observed that as the disease progressed, so the zones moved from proximal to distal until the entire scaphoid was osteonecrotic. They proposed a classification based on the chronologic stage of the disease as the disease progresses from proximal to distal. They also noted fractures in 80% of the patients they reviewed. These fractures were all in the proximal pole of the scaphoid and were never transverse in relation to the longitudinal axis of the scaphoid.

Computerized tomography

Computerized tomography (CT) imaging of the affected scaphoid may be useful to identify areas of scaphoid fragmentation, cyst formation, deformity, and fracture as well as associated carpal instability (**Figs. 3**B and **4**B). We have also recently used 4D (dynamic) CT scans to better understand this condition. It demonstrates the fragmentation and the "internal instability" within the scaphoid, where different parts of the scaphoid move independently, creating a carpal instability (Video 1).

Arthroscopy

Arthroscopic assessment of Kienbock's disease is well established[18,19] and can help guide appropriate treatment. Arthroscopic assessment and

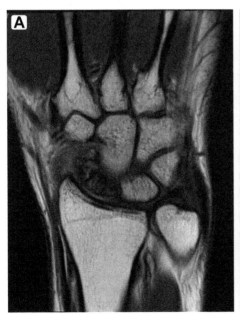
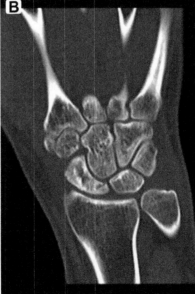

Fig. 2. The right wrist of a 32-year-old woman. (*A*) MRI demonstrating Type 1 Kalainov Preiser's disease with involvement of the entire scaphoid. (*B*) CT scan demonstrating fragmentation and fracture of the scaphoid and evidence of carpal instability—See also Video 1. (*Courtesy of* Dr. Gregory Bain, South Australia, Australia.)

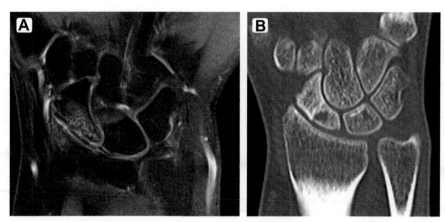

Fig. 3. The right wrist of a 35-year-old woman. (*A*) MRI scan demonstrating Type 2 Kalainov Preiser's disease with only part of the scaphoid affected. (*B*) CT scan demonstrating fragmentation and fracture in the longitudinal plan of the proximal pole of the scaphoid. (*Courtesy of* Simon MacLean, MBChB, FRCS(Tr&Orth), PGDipCE, Bay of Plenty, New Zealand.)

subsequent treatment of Preiser's disease, however, are confined to case reports.[20–22] Arthroscopy may be diagnostic and therapeutic and is the gold standard in assessing the status of the articular surfaces of the scaphoid and remainder of the carpus. In early stages of the disease, the chondral surfaces may be intact. Probe ballottement allows assessment of the integrity of the underlying subchondral bone plate. Synovitis may be present, and an arthroscopic synovectomy may be performed. The status of the remaining chondral surfaces in the wrist can be evaluated. Intrinsic ligaments of the wrist can be assessed. In cases of scaphoid fracture and fragmentation, an arthroscopic debridement can be performed.

Possible Etiology

By definition, the cause of an idiopathic condition is unknown; it is also possible that the cause is multifactorial and that there are anatomic, vascular, mechanical, and/or biological factors that contribute to the development of the disease.

The blood supply to the scaphoid has been well described. Preiser was the first to describe it using injection techniques and radiographs to visualize the arterial blood supply and described how the majority of the scaphoid's blood supply entered from the radial artery on the dorsal aspect of the scaphoid (**Fig. 1**C, D). 70 years after this description, Gelberman and colleagues[23] described how the blood supply to the scaphoid enters via nonarticular areas of ligamentous attachments in branches from the radial artery. The proximal 70% to 80% of the scaphoid receives its blood supply from a branch entering via the dorsal ridge while the tuberosity and distal 20% to 30% of the

scaphoid receives its blood from the volar radial artery and volar palmar arch. There is no anastomosis between these two supplies meaning damage to the main dorsal blood supply cannot be adequately compensated for. This probably explains why Preiser's disease predominantly affects the proximal pole that has a relatively poor blood supply.

Butterman and colleagues[24] further examined the blood supply to the scaphoid in a cadaveric model and found that arterioles pass through an intra-articular membrane between the wrist capsule and the dorsal ridge and that these may be at risk of damage from increased intra-articular pressures. In the same cadaveric study, they examined the extrinsic pressure created by the extensor carpi radialis brevis (ECRB) tendon as it passes over the dorsal ridge of the scaphoid and found a significant increase in pressure created by flexion of 60° to 90° and 15° of ulna deviation of the wrist.

Butterman postulated that the etiology of scaphoid avascular necrosis was repetitive wrist loading creating a secondary wrist effusion, which obstructs the delicate arterioles, as they supply to the dorsal scaphoid. Kienbocks disease is thought to occur in 'at-risk' patients, with 'at-risk' lunate in an 'at-risk region' of the lunate. With repetitive loading, a stress fracture occurs in the subchondral bone occluding the subarticular venous plexus, which results in venous hypertension, intraosseous compartment syndrome, and subsequently avascular necrosis.[25] It is possible that there is a similar etiology and pathogenesis for Preiser's disease, but the natural history of the disease is not sufficiently understood to have identified these 'at-risk' factors in Preiser's disease.

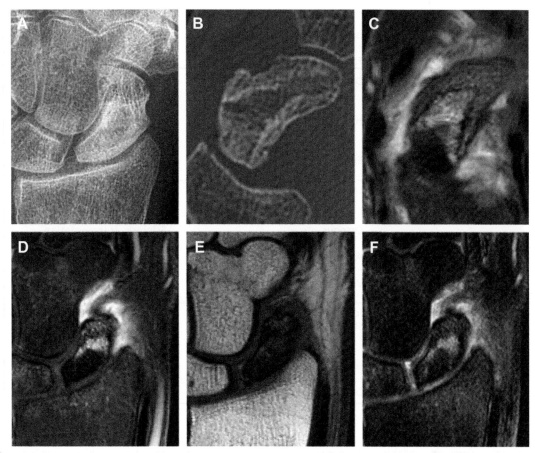

Fig. 4. A 60-year-old woman suffering from Preiser's disease of the left scaphoid. (*A*) The dorsopalmar radiograph shows narrowing (nipple sign) and increased bone density of the proximal scaphoid pole. (*B*) Sagittal-oblique CT scan reveals a tiny cortical fragment at the palmar side of the proximal pole additionally to zones of different bone density. (*C*) In the sagittal-oblique MRI (contrast-enhanced T1 SE with fat-suppression), a three-layered architecture of the scaphoid in Preiser's disease is evident. (*D–F*) Coronal MRI (d = fat-saturated PD FSE, e = unenhanced T1 SE, and f = contrast-enhanced and fat-saturated T1 SE) allows to differentiate three layers of the scaphoid in Preiser's diseases. The proximal zone is nonviable (without bone marrow edema and without contrast enhancement), the middle zone is hyperemic and hypervascular, and residual normal bone marrow is maintained in the distal zone. (*From* Schmitt R, Fröhner S, van Schoonhoven J, Lanz U, Gölles A. Idiopathic osteonecrosis of the scaphoid (Preiser's disease)–MRI gives new insights into etiology and pathology. Eur J Radiol. 2011;77(2):228-234. https://doi.org/10.1016/j.ejrad.2010.11.009; with pemission.)

Management

The choice of management of Preiser's disease is controversial. The natural history remains poorly understood, but we do know that the disease occurs along a spectrum from isolated scaphoid pathology to advanced carpal collapse. The associated pain may range from minor to debilitating. Therefore, management should be based on specific treatment aims.

Aims of treatment

The aims of treatment are to:

1. Improve the patient's pain.

2. Protect the scaphoid from collapse.
3. Protect the wrist joint from collapse and degeneration.
4. If the scaphoid is compromised, consider reconstruction
5. If the scaphoid is not reconstructible, or the wrist is unstable or degenerate, consider a motion-preserving reconstructive procedure.
6. If the wrist is not reconstructible, consider a salvage procedure.

Factors for consideration There are many factors to consider in individualizing the management plan including patient characteristics and the state of the scaphoid and carpus (**Table 2**).

Table 2
Factors to consider in planning management

	Factors- 2	Factors - 3
Patient	Demographics	Age, sex, occupation, activities, comorbidities, medications, smoking
	History	Injury, pain, aggravating factors, duration of symptoms
	Examination	Swelling, tenderness, range of motion, grip strength
Scaphoid	Loading	Morphology of the carpus, ulnar variance, radial inclination
	Osseous	Sclerosis, fragmentation, collapse
	Articular	Functional articulations, lamination, degeneration
	Vascularity	Ischemia, necrosis, revascularization
Wrist	Joint	Synovitis, contracture
	Stability	Carpal collapse (RSA > 60), scapholunate and lunotriquetral tears, radial translocation of the distal carpal row
	Degeneration	Localized, generalized

After considering these factors, the following treatment options are available to the surgeon;

Nonoperative treatment

- We recommend a combination of splinting, activity modification, analgesics, and non-steroidal anti-inflammatory drugs (NSAID's) at the time of presentation. Although some authors have reported some good results for nonoperative treatments,[26] most authors report progression of disease with conservative treatment.[27–29] Video 1 demonstrates progressive fragmentation of the Preiser's scaphoid, with significant reabsorption and associated carpal instability with radial translation of the distal carpal row seen.

Unloading

- Radial closing wedge osteotomy (CRWO)—Tomori et al.[30] described seven patients in which two patients also had concomitant Kienbocks disease. They reported improved pain and range of motion in all patients and even improved vascularization on MRI scan. However, four patients had radiographic progression and collapse of the scaphoid. The original authors rationale for this was that

they had noted increased radial inclination, and that this procedure would function to shift the loading of the wrist away from the affected scaphoid.
- It is possible that this joint leveling procedure has the effect of changing the loading vector on the affected scaphoid—which may be protective, decreasing the local joint reaction forces, and that surgery near the affected scaphoid creates a localized hyperemic effect improving the local blood supply to the affected scaphoid.
- We would therefore consider the use of a CRWO when there is a significant increase in radial inclination with an intact scaphoid.

Reconstruction

- Vascularized bone grafts (VBGs)—Pronator quadratus pedicled VBGs[15,31,32] 1,2 or 2,3 Intercompartmental artery supra-retinacular artery vascularized grafts[33] have been described for Herbert stage 2 disease cases. From these studies of 18 patients, most had good to excellent outcomes and evidence of revascularization on MRI in all cases (though incomplete to the proximal pole in some). Despite these improvements, three patients

Table 3
Authors approach to Preiser's disease

Scaphoid	Treatment	Comment
Intact	Diagnostic arthroscopy and debridement	If increased radial inclination = consider CRWO
Fragmented and/or collapsed	Motion preserving procedure (PRC OR three-corner fusion)	Intact midcarpal articulation, >40 y, low demand = consider PRC. <40 years, high demand = three-corner fusion
	Salvage (arthrodesis or arthroplasty)	Reserved for failed surgery

develop arthritis with one requiring revision surgery to a proximal row carpectomy (PRC).

- We feel that any attempted revascularization procedures should be reserved for cases before scaphoid fragmentation, collapse, or instability. Use of VBGs in scaphoid nonunion and avascular necrosis after trauma is controversial,[34,35] and its use in Presiers disease is unknown. We have not performed a VBG in a patient with Preiser's disease. From our experience in Kienbock's Disease, our rationale remains the same however, and we believe any attempted revascularization procedure should be combined with *temporary unloading of the graft* using a buried lunocapitate K-wire for 10 to 12 weeks.

Motion preserving

- Surgical debridement—both open[26] and arthroscopic debridement[20,22] of the affected area of the scaphoid have been described with good results reported even with Herbert Stage 3 disease. Debridement of radiocarpal and midcarpal synovitis, loose bodies, and fragmented scaphoid can be performed arthroscopically and offers a lower morbidity approach than open procedures so is our preference. It also facilitates accurate assessment of the adjacent distant carpal articulations for further treatment planning.
- Proximal row carpectomy—De Smet and colleagues[36] reported on the use of PRC in the management of 12 patients with Preiser's disease, He reported 10 were satisfied, with a mean visual analogue scale (VAS) score of 0, grip strength of 18.9 kg, and mean flexion/extension of nearly 75°. A single patient 'in doubt' and a single patient dissatisfied who had conversion to total wrist replacement.
- Limited wrist fusions—there are only a handful of partial wrist fusions reported in the literature with varying results. We have used the three-

corner fusion for some of these cases.[37] This is performed by excising the fragmented scaphoid and fusing the lunate-capitate-hamate articulation. The excised triquetrum provides a good bone graft, reduces the chance of ulnar carpal impaction, and increases the range of motion.[38]

We consider the use of PRC and limited wrist fusion in a similar way to their use in scaphoid nonunion advanced collapse (SNAC). Arthroscopic assessment before these procedures is an excellent adjunct.

Salvage

- Partial wrist replacement—Scaphoid excision and silastic implant have been reported[5,26] with mixed results; at medium-term follow-up, good results have been seen but these have not lasted with residual pain, weakness, and decreased range of motion in the longer term. Arthroscopic surgical debridement of the entire proximal pole with subsequent pyrocarbon implant has been described[21] with good preliminary results in terms of pain relief but minimal improvement in stiffness and no follow-up beyond 6 months.
- Total wrist replacement or fusion—While these have been described in some cases of Preiser's disease, it has been in patients where other surgical interventions have failed and no outcomes have been reported.
- We would recommend the use of these options only as salvage procedures when other options have failed and not as a first-line treatment.

Authors approach to Preiser's disease
We prefer to assess Preiser's disease using 4D CT, contrast MRI, and arthroscopy. This allows us to assess the scaphoid, any associated carpal instability and the rest of the wrist. Our preferred treatment options are summarized in **Table 3**.

SUMMARY

The term Preiser's disease has been used to describe avascular necrosis of the scaphoid due to a number of causes, but mostly it is described as being idiopathic. It is rare and the natural history is not fully understood. Management of the condition should be based on patient factors as well as the stage of disease within the scaphoid and the surrounding wrist. This chapter appraises the available evidence and aims to provide the reader with a framework to manage this rare condition.

DISCLOSURE

The authors declare no conflicts of interest.

SUPPLEMENTARY DATA

Supplementary data to this article can be found online at https://doi.org/10.1016/j.hcl.2022.03.013.

REFERENCES

1. Preiser G. Eine typische posttraumatische und zur Spontanfraktur führende Ostitis des Naviculare carpi. Fortschr Röntgenstr 1910;15:189–97.
2. Preiser G. Zur Frage der typischen traumatischen Ernährungs- störungen der kurzen Hand- und Fusswurzelknochen. Fortschr Röntgenstr 1911;17:360–2.
3. Kallen AM, Strackee SD. On the history and definition of Preiser's disease. J Hand Surg Eur Vol 2014;39(7):770–6.
4. Preiser G. Zur Frage der typischen traumatischen Ernährungs- störungen der kurzen Hand- und Fusswurzelknochen. Fortschr Röntgenstr 1911;17:360–2.
5. Herbert TJ, Lanzetta M. Idiopathic avascular necrosis of the scaphoid. J Hand Surg Br 1994;19(2): 174–82.
6. Ferlic DC, Morin P. Idiopathic avascular necrosis of the scaphoid: Preiser's disease? J Hand Surg Am 1989;14(1):13–6.
7. Bray TJ, McCarroll HR Jr. Preiser's disease: a case report. J Hand Surg Am 1984;9(5):730–2.
8. Chang CC, Greenspan A, Gershwin ME. Osteonecrosis: current perspectives on pathogenesis and treatment. Semin Arthritis Rheum 1993;23(1):47–69.
9. Kawai H, Tsuyuguchi Y, Yonenobu K, et al. Avascular necrosis of the carpal scaphoid associated with progressive systemic sclerosis. Hand 1983;15(3): 270–3.
10. Virik K, Karapetis C, Droufakou S, et al. Avascular necrosis of bone: the hidden risk of glucocorticoids used as antiemetics in cancer chemotherapy. Int J Clin Pract 2001;55(5):344–5.
11. Aptekar RG, Klippel JH, Becker KE, et al. Avascular necrosis of the talus, scaphoid, and metatarsal head in systemic lupus erythematosus. Clin Orthop Relat Res 1974;101:127–8.
12. Harper PG, Trask C, Souhami RL. Avascular necrosis of bone caused by combination chemotherapy without corticosteroids. Br Med J (Clin Res Ed) 1984;288(6413):267–8.
13. Tate DE, Gupta A, Kleinert HE. Bipartite scaphoid with proximal pole osteonecrosis in a patient with Holt-Oram syndrome. J Hand Surg Br 2000;25(1): 112–4.
14. Bergman S, Petit A, Rabarin F, et al. Preiser's disease or avascular osteonecrosis of the scaphoid: An updated literature review. Hand Surg Rehabil 2021;40(4):359–68.
15. Lenoir H, Coulet B, Lazerges C, et al. Idiopathic avascular necrosis of the scaphoid: 10 new cases and a review of the literature. Indications for Preiser's disease. Orthop Traumatol Surg Res 2012;98(4): 390–7.
16. Kalainov DM, Cohen MS, Hendrix RW, et al. Preiser's disease: identification of two patterns. J Hand Surg Am 2003;28(5):767–78.
17. Schmitt R, Fröhner S, van Schoonhoven J, et al. Idiopathic osteonecrosis of the scaphoid (Preiser's disease)–MRI gives new insights into etiology and pathology. Eur J Radiol 2011;77(2):228–34.
18. Bain GI, Begg M. Arthroscopic assessment and classification of Kienbock's disease. Tech Hand Up Extrem Surg 2006;10(1):8–13.
19. Bain GI, MacLean SB, Tse WL, et al. Kienböck disease and arthroscopy: assessment, classification, and treatment. J Wrist Surg 2016;5(4):255–60.
20. Menth-Chiari WA, Poehling GG. Preiser's disease: arthroscopic treatment of avascular necrosis of the scaphoid. Arthroscopy 2000;16(2):208–13.
21. Rousseau B, Delpit X, Bauer T, et al. Maladie de Preiser traitée par résection partielle du scaphoïde sous arthroscopie et implant en pyrocarbone, résultats préliminaires : à propos d'un cas, et revue de la littérature [Arthroscopic treatment for Preiser's disease by partial resection of the scaphoid and pyrocarbone's implant, preliminary results: a case report and literature review]. Chir Main 2011;30(3): 231–5. French.
22. Viegas SF. Arthroscopic treatment of osteochondritis dissecans of the scaphoid. Arthroscopy 1988;4(4): 278–81.
23. Gelberman RH, Menon J. The vascularity of the scaphoid bone. J Hand Surg Am 1980;5(5):508–13.
24. Buttermann GR, Putnam MD, Shine JD. Wrist position affects loading of the dorsal scaphoid: possible effect on extrinsic scaphoid blood flow. J Hand Surg Br 2001;26(1):34–40.
25. Bain GI, MacLean SB, Yeo CJ, et al. The Etiology and Pathogenesis of Kienböck Disease [published correction appears in J Wrist Surg. 2016 Nov;5(4): e1]. J Wrist Surg 2016;5(4):248–54.

26. Vidal MA, Linscheid RL, Amadio PC, et al. Preiser's disease. Ann Chir Main Memb Super 1991;10(3): 227–35.

27. Lauder AJ, Trumble TE. Idiopathic avascular necrosis of the scaphoid: Preiser's disease. Hand Clin 2006;22(4):475–vi.

28. El Kouhen F, Gay AM, Chateau F, et al. La maladie de Preiser : une série de cinq cas [Preiser's disease: a five-case series]. Chir Main 2012;31(1):45–51.

29. Tomori Y, Nanno M, Takai S. Clinical outcomes of nonsurgical treatment for Preiser disease. Medicine (Baltimore) 2020;99(4):e18883.

30. Tomori Y, Sawaizumi T, Nanno M, et al. Closing radial wedge osteotomy for preiser disease: clinical outcomes. J Hand Surg Am 2019;44(10):896.e1–10.

31. Hou S, Liu T. Pronator quadratus pedicled bone graft for idiopathic avascular necrosis of the scaphoid. Orthop Int Ed 1994;2:267–9.

32. Kara T, Gunal I. Preiser's disease treated by pronotor quadratus pedicled bone graft. J Plast Surg Hand Surg 2014;48(6):455–6.

33. Moran SL, Cooney WP, Shin AY. The use of vascularized grafts from the distal radius for the treatment of Preiser's disease. J Hand Surg Am 2006;31(5):705–10.

34. Pinder RM, Brkljac M, Rix L, et al. Treatment of scaphoid nonunion: a systematic review of the existing evidence. J Hand Surg Am 2015;40(9):1797–805. e3.

35. Ferguson DO, Shanbhag V, Hedley H, et al. Scaphoid fracture non-union: a systematic review of surgical treatment using bone graft. J Hand Surg Eur Vol 2016;41(5):492–500.

36. de Smet L. Avascular nontraumatic necrosis of the scaphoid. Preiser's disease? Chir Main 2000;19(2): 82–5.

37. van Riet RP, Bain GI. Three-corner wrist fusion using memory staples. Tech Hand Up Extrem Surg 2006; 10(4):259–64.

38. Bain GI, Sood A, Ashwood N, et al. Effect of scaphoid and triquetrum excision after limited stabilisation on cadaver wrist movement. J Hand Surg Eur Vol 2009;34(5):614–7.

Avascular Necrosis of Capitate and Other Uncommon Presentations of Carpal Avascular Necrosis

Brent B. Pickrell, MD,
Carl M. Harper, MD, Assistant Professor of Orthopedic Surgery*

KEYWORDS

- Avascular necrosis (AVN) • Capitate AVN • Carpal bone AVN • Uncommon carpal bone AVN

KEY POINTS

- Avascular necrosis (AVN) of the individual carpal bones is an uncommon cause of wrist pain and disability.
- Owing to the rarity of these disease processes, a high index suspicion is required to make the diagnosis in addition to use of advanced imaging and/or arthroscopy.
- Owing to the paucity of comparative studies and long-term outcomes data, there is currently little evidence to guide management.

INTRODUCTION

Avascular necrosis (AVN) of an individual carpal bone is an uncommon cause of wrist pain and disability. Owing to incompletely understood etiopathogenesis, certain carpal bones are more susceptible to AVN than the others. While AVN of the lunate and scaphoid are reported most frequently, AVN of each carpal bone has been described.[1] The etiology of AVN of the carpal bones is thought to be multifactorial, with prior studies citing both intrinsic and extrinsic factors, including trauma, bone morphology, and vascular predisposition and/or injury.[2]

DIAGNOSIS

Owing to the rarity of these disease processes, a high index of suspicion is required to make the diagnosis. Frequently, a patient will present with insidious onset of wrist pain and stiffness with no history of trauma. Swelling, tenderness, diminished grip strength, and decreased range of motion (ROM) are common, albeit nonspecific, findings.

Imaging should be universally pursued as a part of the initial workup. Standard radiographs in the setting of AVN may seem unremarkable in the early stages of the disease process. However, given that these pathologies are frequently missed, it is not uncommon for patients to present with late-stage disease and evidence of sclerosis, fragmentation, cyst formation, fracture, carpal collapse, and even secondary arthritic changes on initial radiograph.[3]

In the early stages of AVN, plain radiographs are often normal. Contrast-enhanced magnetic resonance imaging (MRI) with gadolinium is more sensitive and specific to demonstrate bone marrow edema and involvement. In the early stage, T1-weighted MRI demonstrates low signal intensity, whereas T2-weighted MRI demonstrates increased signal intensity. Later through the AVN process, decreased signal intensity on T2-weighted MRI may denote a worse prognosis.[3]

CAPITATE AVN

After AVN of the scaphoid and lunate, AVN of the capitate is the third most commonly reported

Department of Orthopedic Surgery, 330 Brookline Avenue–Stoneman 10, Boston, MA 02215, USA
* Corresponding author.
E-mail address: charper@bidmc.harvard.edu

Hand Clin 38 (2022) 479–485
https://doi.org/10.1016/j.hcl.2022.03.009

AVN within the carpus. Capitate AVN may involve part or all of the head, distal body, or the entire bone.[4]

Capitate AVN is most often secondary to trauma[5,6] and has been reported in the setting of perilunate "greater arc" injuries, including the rare scaphocapitate fracture variant (naviculo-capitate fracture syndrome).[7] This injury pattern is characterized by transverse fractures of both the scaphoid and capitate with subsequent rotation of the proximal capitate up to 180°.[8,9] Repetitive minor trauma has also been described.[10–15] Nontraumatic etiologies/associations, such as steroid use,[5,16–19] systemic lupus erythematosus,[20] gout,[5,21] hematologic malignancy,[18] dorsal instability,[22] and certain lysosomal storage diseases,[23,24] have also been implicated. In contrast to the idiopathic variant of scaphoid and lunate AVN, idiopathic capitate AVN, first reported by Jönsson in 1942,[25] remains a rare diagnosis and is most commonly reported in women and younger patients.[5] To date, only 2 cases of bilateral capitate AVN have been described.[18,26]

Similar to the lunate and scaphoid, the capitate receives its blood supply from nutrient vessels that course retrograde within the bone after entering at the distal pole. An early anatomic study identified a retrograde blood supply to the proximal pole of the capitate in all 10 cadaver specimens.[27,28] As such, many have attributed capitate AVN to its predisposing anatomy, analogous to the pathophysiology of scaphoid nonunion. However, several authors have recently challenged this notion, citing a low incidence of capitate AVN following capitate-shortening osteotomy for Kienbock disease.[29,30] Moreover, a recent study using three-dimensional micro-CT[29] noted that 70% of capitate specimens also had at least one vessel directly supplying the proximal pole through the volar capitate ligaments. Despite this newer evidence, many of the current mechanistic explanations for capitate AVN directly or indirectly implicate its intraosseous anatomy.[1,18,20,31,32]

Similar to other carpal AVN, diagnosis is suspected based on history, physical examination, and imaging studies. A recent review found that nearly all published cases of capitate AVN presented with chronic dorsal wrist pain with use/loading, reduced ROM, stiffness, and swelling.[5] The average age at diagnosis was 27 years, with symptoms having been present for 1.7 years (range: 0.1–14) before diagnosis.[5] Radiographic signs included sclerosis and cyst formation along with capitate and carpal collapse.[5] Diagnosis can be further supported with MRI, particularly in the early stages of disease when radiographic findings may be subtle or absent.[18,28,33] Low signal

intensity on T1-weighted images seems to be the most reliable indicator of the presence of AVN.[34] Additionally, arthroscopy may be a useful adjunct to allow direct visualization of the midcarpal space and the individual articular surfaces for treatment planning purposes.[31,35,36]

Milliez and Peters[4,5] proposed a radiographic classification system based on the location of capitate involvement (**Box 1**). In a comprehensive literature review, the Milliez type 1 pattern was found to be most common.[5] Although descriptive in nature, the Milliez classification system does not offer treatment guidelines or prognostic information.

TREATMENT OF CAPITATE AVN

In early stages of capitate AVN, nonsurgical treatments may be considered, including immobilization, anti-inflammatory medication, and activity modification.[37] Some advocate for this approach given that some degree of spontaneous revascularization of the capitate is possible, particularly in younger patients.[28] This has been demonstrated both histologically and on arteriography.[28] However, despite some early reports of successful outcomes,[5,15] conservative management seems to yield inconsistent results.[16,18,20,23,37,38]

Surgical treatment should be considered in patients that fail nonoperative management or present with more advanced disease, particularly carpal fragmentation and collapse. Previously reported surgical procedures include open proximal pole resection,[11,38] partial arthroscopic resection,[35] capitate excision with prosthetic[26,39] or autologous soft-tissue interposition arthroplasty,[33,38] vascularized or nonvascularized bone grafting,[5,11,13,18,28,34,39–45] limited intercarpal fusion,[5,17,21,26,27,31,32,36,46,47] four-corner fusion,[5,18] total-wrist fusion,[33] and wrist denervation.[36,40] Selecting the appropriate surgical therapy depends on accurate assessment of the

---

Box 1
Milliez Classification of Capitate AVN

Type I: AVN of the proximal pole
- 1a: dome-shaped central lesion
- 1b: total head and neck
- 1c: radioproximal portion

Type II: AVN of the distal body

Type III: AVN of entire capitate

Data from Walker LG. Avascular necrosis of the capitate. J Hand Surg Am. 1993 Nov;18(6):1129.

bony extent of AVN and the integrity of the adjacent midcarpal joint surfaces.[36] Even then, there is no established surgical treatment protocol for capitate AVN given the paucity of high-quality comparative studies.[5] Unfortunately, long-term outcomes for the various reported surgical procedures are also limited, precluding an evidence-based approach to management.

In the presence of preserved carpal height and uninvolved midcarpal articular surface(s), some authors argue that the chosen intervention should preserve the midcarpal space.[31] As such, debridement with or without cancellous or vascularized bone graft (VBG) may be considered.[40] Ichchou and colleagues[40] reported excision of the necrotic capitate along with corticocancellous graft from the olecranon in a young female patient with idiopathic AVN. The patient was reportedly pain-free in short-term follow-up. Murakami[11,28] also reported good outcomes following curettage, drilling, and iliac crest bone grafting. However, in their review, Peters and colleagues[5] noted that the results of nonvascularized bone grafting were unsatisfactory, with 3 patients experiencing "fair" to "good" results and 2 with "poor" results. There has since been another report of nonvascularized corticocancellous iliac crest graft in a pediatric patient who thereafter achieved full-wrist ROM and no pain at 2-year follow-up.[39] In contrast, reports of local VBG from the distal radius and metacarpals have offered more optimistic outcomes. Imai and colleagues[41] reported a case of VBG from the distal radius based on the 2,3-intercompartmental supraretinacular artery. Two years postoperatively, the patient recovered full ROM and grip strength was 23 kg (from 4 kg) compared with 25 kg of the contralateral side. The authors noted that the long arc of the pedicle provided adequate length to fill the entirety of the capitate. Utilizing the fourth extensor compartment artery (ECA), Hattori and colleagues[13] reported a case of VBG in a high-school baseball pitcher who had preservation of his proximal articular surface. To increase unloading of the capitate during the healing process, the authors also placed an external fixator for 8 weeks. At 1-year follow-up, the patient reported no pain and was able to resume pitching. Similarly, Strauss and colleagues,[18] in a report of bilateral capitate AVN, were able to successfully utilize a unilateral 4,5-ECA VBG to revascularize a capitate with an intact proximal articular surface. Immobilization was maintained postoperatively using a dorsal spanning plate that was removed after 2 months, at which time the patient was noted to be pain-free. Bekele and colleagues[34] also reported use of the 4,5-ECA VBG but instead temporarily unloaded the capitate with K-wires placed

from the distal scaphoid into the distal capitate. Vascularized bone from the base of the second metacarpal in the setting of proximal pole (type 1) AVN has also been described.[42] At 14-month follow-up, the patient had achieved normal grip strength (16 kg from 4 kg) and improvement in visual analog scale (VAS) and Mayo Wrist scores. Among the several advantages of the second metacarpal VBG noted by the authors was the consistent anatomy of the first dorsal metacarpal artery. Finally, microvascular bone transfer in the form of iliac crest[43] and medial femoral condyle (MFC) flaps[44] has also been described. Bürger and colleagues[43] reported use of a free vascularized iliac crest bone graft to preserve the proximal pole of the capitate in a 19-year-old male athlete. Kazmers and colleagues[44] described a case in a 16-year-old female patient with an intact proximal articular surface who underwent curettage and MFC flap reconstruction. The patient returned to all normal activities by 6 months after surgery. At the final follow-up at 18 months, the patient remained pain-free, continued unrestricted activities, and had attained normal grip strength. The authors cite that, if the proximal articulation had been found to be involved intraoperatively, the versatility of the genicular arterial tree can permit harvest of an osteocartilaginous flap (ie, medial femoral trochlear [MFT] flap) instead.

Alternatively, when patients present with proximal articular involvement with concomitant collapse, resection/debridement alone or combined with interposition arthroplasty has been successfully used. Proximal capitate excision and interposition arthroplasty first included individual reports of soft-tissue interposition using a fourth toe extensor tendon or palmaris longus tendon.[33,38] In the former report, the patient went on to have persistent pain 6 months after her extensor tendon interposition and eventually required a wrist arthrodesis. However, in the latter report, the patient was able to return to her job as a typist 10 months after surgery and reported only mild pain.[38] The most recent report[39] includes a case of pyrocarbon interposition arthroplasty in a 15-year-old rugby player who became pain-free 6 weeks following surgery. At 1 year postoperatively, he had successfully returned to rugby, and at the time of the final follow-up (3.5 years), he had been working full-time as a construction plant mechanic for 2 years where he was performing regular heavy lifting. Successful use of a silicone prosthesis following excision of the capitate head had been previously reported by Bolton-Maggs and colleagues.[26] Alternatively, autologous replacement of the proximal articular surface is possible. One previous publication described use of the MFT flap for proximal articular surface replacement in a 28-year-old patient with idiopathic proximal AVN and preserved distal lunate cartilage.[45]

Technical refinements in wrist arthroscopy have also engendered new treatment options. Shimizu and colleagues[35] reported a series of 5 patients with cystic changes and collapse at the proximal pole (Milliez type Ia) that underwent successful arthroscopic resection of the capitate head and lunate facet. All patients achieved pain relief and improved wrist ROM and grip strength following their procedure. At the latest follow-up, the mean wrist flexion–extension was 123° (from 81° preoperatively) and grip strength was 74% (from 37% preoperatively). The VAS pain score (6.8–1.1), Disabilities of the Arm, Shoulder, and Hand (DASH) score (40–12), and Patient-Rated Wrist Evaluation score (59–19) all showed significant improvement following treatment. Postoperative radiographic parameters showed no significant changes of carpal malalignment or evidence of midcarpal arthritis at an average follow-up of 20 months.

When the midcarpal joint has chondral lesions involving the scaphocapitate and/or lunocapitate joints, and/or when capitate fragmentation and/or collapse is present, consideration for intercarpal arthrodesis is appropriate. This is often combined with cancellous bone grafting to optimize bone healing potential.[5,46] Of the different midcarpal arthrodesis options for capitate AVN, the scaphocapitolunate (SCL) arthrodesis has been reported most frequently.[5] Vander Grend and colleagues[27] reported early success on 2 patients with carpal collapse managed with SCL arthrodesis with subsequent relief of symptoms. Similarly, De Smet and colleagues[21] reported success in a patient with advanced midcarpal arthritis and capitate AVN in the setting of gout. Arcalis Arce and colleagues[32] reported a case of idiopathic capitate AVN in a male carpenter who was able to return to his job unimpeded following SCL arthrodesis. Whiting and Rotman[47] also reported on SCL arthrodesis in conjunction with corticocancellous bone graft from the iliac crest to restore carpal height in a young female. At 1 year postoperatively, grip and pinch strength were both improved and the patient endorsed resolution of her pain. In 2015, Peters and colleagues[5] reported on 4 patients with proximal (type 1) capitate AVN with and without carpal collapse who underwent SLC arthrodesis with autologous bone grafting and an average follow-up of 9 years. Three of the 4 patients were satisfied with the procedure and demonstrated improved VAS, DASH, and Mayo Wrist scores. One patient went on to have residual pain at a degenerative triquetrum–hamate joint,

and this resulted in the need to change vocation. Most recently, Athlani and colleagues[36] reported a series of 5 patients with arthroscopically proven midcarpal arthritis managed with SCL arthrodesis and cancellous bone grafting with a mean 5-year follow-up. Fusion was achieved in 100%, and all patients experienced functional improvement, including grip strength (averaging 90% of contralateral side). No patients had evidence of midcarpal collapse at the latest follow-up.

Other reported arthrodesis techniques include capitolunate,[17] capitohamate,[31] 4-corner arthrodesis,[5,18] and even multiple intercarpal fusions.[26,46] Ansari and colleagues[31] reported a case of type 3 AVN with midcarpal joint space narrowing that was treated with capitate hemiresection followed by capitohamate fusion and a distally based extensor carpi radialis longus tendon interposition. One year after surgery, the patient was asymptomatic and had radiographic evidence of fusion with maintenance of the midcarpal space. In their series, Peters and colleagues[5] also reported 2 cases with carpal collapse that were treated with 4-corner fusion with fair results, including 1 incomplete fusion of the hamate. The authors noted that pain may persist at sites of incomplete fusion and advised meticulous preparation of the arthrodesis sites and the impaction of cancellous bone to optimize bone healing. In a case of staggered bilateral capitate AVN, Strauss and colleagues[18] initially undertook 4-corner fusion with a circular plate in a 25-year-old female patient. At the 3-month follow-up visit, the patient reported complete resolution of pain. At 18 months postoperatively, her flexion/extension arc was 50°/50° compared with 85°/85° on the contralateral wrist that underwent a pedicled VBG from the distal radius. Overall, intercarpal arthrodesis seems to provide good pain relief but also loss of motion and grip strength; however, these appear well tolerated.[5] Failed limited intercarpal fusions and those patients presenting with significant preoperative carpal collapse should be considered for 4-corner arthrodesis.

Salvage surgeries for capitate AVN include total-wrist arthrodesis and wrist denervation.[48] Leonard and Mullet[48] presented a case of a 16-year-old female with idiopathic capitate AVN that failed conservative management and underwent successful posterior interosseous nerve (PIN) neurectomy. By 4 weeks postoperatively, her rest pain had resolved, and at 2-year follow-up, she had regained an almost full ROM in her wrist. Radiographs revealed sclerosis but no collapse. Walker[14] also presented a case of a similarly aged female gymnast who underwent successful PIN neurectomy and demonstrated satisfaction with her wrist function, ROM, and comfort level at 1-year follow-up. Partial wrist denervation can also be combined with other procedures. Using a dorsal approach, Ichchou and colleagues[40] combined PIN neurectomy with corticoconcellous grafting in a patient with idiopathic AVN who was pain-free at 2-month follow-up.

AVN OF OTHER CARPAL BONES

AVN of the remaining carpal bones is even more rare, with most published studies existing in the form of isolated case reports. Given their overall rarity, it is impossible to formulate a meaningful classification system or treatment algorithm with which to guide management. A recent review[3] outlines the individual case reports and case series with respect to each carpal AVN.

Only four cases of triquetral AVN have been reported in the literature.[49–52] Previous reports have implicated trauma, local steroid injections, and heavy smoking. One case[49] responded to conservative measures, whereas the others did not.[50–52] In the most recent report,[52] proximal row carpectomy (PRC) provided sufficient relief of symptoms in a patient with a significant smoking history. Given the success, longevity, and relative technical ease of PRC in treating multiple wrist pathologies involving the proximal carpal row, PRC seems well suited to treat triquetral AVN in the authors' opinion.

AVN of the trapezium has been reported three times.[53–55] One case had normalization on MRI following 3 months of conservative treatment with casting and anti-inflammatory medication.[54] A second case[55] was treated with a 1,2-intercompartmental supraretinacular artery VBG from the distal radius and had good outcomes at 1 year postoperatively. A third case[53] was treated successfully with trapezial resection and suspension arthroplasty using a partial flexor carpi radialis interposition graft. Given the success of trapezial resection (with or without tendon interposition) in treating CMC arthritis, this would be the authors' first line of treatment following failure of conservative management.

AVN of the trapezoid has been reported four times,[56–59] including one case of bilateral involvement[56] and one case recently reported in an adolescent.[58] Another case[59] developed 3 months following CMC arthroplasty and resolved with immobilization. Two other cases[56,58] were also treated satisfactorily without operations, including the aforementioned patient with bilateral trapezoid AVN. Another case failed a trial of conservative treatment and ultimately underwent curettage, iliac crest bone graft, and core revascularization using the dorsal metacarpal vascular bundle.[57]

AVN of the pisiform has been reported three times.[60–62] The rarity is not surprising given the relatively rich vascularity of the pisiform, as evidenced by its use as a VBG for treatment of Kienbock disease.[63–65] Prior authors have opted for pisiform excision.

AVN of the hamate has been reported over a dozen times.[66] Treatment depends on the location of the AVN within the hamate, with the overwhelming majority of prior reports offering some form of surgical treatment to these patients.[66] AVN isolated to the hamate hook seems to respond well to simple excision.[66,67] Other reported treatment options include debridement with cancellous bone grafting,[66,68] VBG from distal radius,[66,69] or some form of intercarpal fusion (capitohamate[70] vs capitolunatohamate[68] vs 4-corner[71]). Interestingly, none of the hamate AVN reports show any carpal collapse on the final follow-up, suggesting that watchful waiting may be an option in select patients who present with tolerable pain.[66]

SUMMARY

In conclusion, outside of Preiser's and Kienbock's disease, AVN of the remaining carpal bones is exceedingly rare with a natural history that is incompletely understood. Most cases present with an insidious onset of wrist pain and dysfunction that may go undiagnosed for months or years, resulting in significant patient morbidity and time away from work. Diagnosis requires a high index of suspicion and advanced imaging; the role of arthroscopy in the diagnosis and treatment of these conditions continues to evolve. Most treatment options aim to debride necrotic bone, promote revascularization (either directly or indirectly), and restore or maintain carpal height.

DISCLOSURE

The authors have nothing to disclose.

REFERENCES

1. Botte MJ, Pacelli LL, Gelberman RH. Vascularity and osteonecrosis of the wrist. Orthop Clin North Am 2004;35(3):405e421.
2. Willems WF, Alberton GM, Bishop AT, et al. Vascularized bone grafting in a canine carpal avascular necrosis model. Clin Orthop Relat Res 2011;469(10): 2831–7.
3. Afshar A, Tabrizi A. Avascular necrosis of the carpal bones other than Kienböck disease. J Hand Surg Am 2020;45(2):148–52.
4. Milliez PY, Kinh Kha H, Allieu Y, et al. Idiopathic aseptic osteonecrosis of the capitate bone.

Literature review apropos of 3 new cases [in French]. Int Orthop 1991;15(2):85–94.

5. Peters SJ, Degreef I, De Smet L. Avascular necrosis of the capitate: report of six cases and review of the literature. J Hand Surg Eur 2015;40(5):520–5.

6. Mansberg R, Lewis G, Kirsh G. Avascular necrosis and fracture of the capitate bone. Clin Nucl Med 2000;25(5):372–3.

7. Fenton RL. The naviculo-capitate fracture syndrome. J Bone Joint Surg Am 1956;38:681–4.

8. Monahan PR, Galasko CS. The scapho-capitate fracture syndrome: a mechanism of injury. J Bone Joint Surg Am 1972;54(1):122–4.

9. Vance RM, Gelberman RH, Evans EF. Scaphocapitate fractures. Patterns of dislocation, mechanisms of injury, and preliminary results of treatment. J Bone Joint Surg Am 1980;62(2):271–6.

10. James ET, Burke FD. Vibration disease of the capitate. J Hand Surg Br 1984;9(2):169–70.

11. Murakami S, Nakajima H. Aseptic necrosis of the capitate bone in two gymnasts. Am J Sports Med 1984;12:170–3.

12. Ye BJ, Kim JI, Lee HJ, et al. A case of avascular necrosis of the capitate bone in a pallet car driver. J Occup Health 2009;51:451–3.

13. Hattori Y, Doi K, Sakamoto S, et al. Vascularized pedicled bone graft for avascular necrosis of the capitate: case report. J Hand Surg Am 2009;34(7):1303–7.

14. Walker LG. Avascular necrosis of the capitate. J Hand Surg Am 1993;18(6):1129.

15. Rahme H. Idiopathic avascular necrosis of the capitate bone–case report. Hand 1983;15(3):274–5.

16. Kato H, Ogino T, Minami A. Steroid-induced avascular necrosis of the capitate: a case report. Handchir Mikrochir Plast Chir 1991;23:15–7.

17. Toker S, Ozer K. Avascular necrosis of the capitate. Orthopedics 2010;33(11):850.

18. Strauss G, Brady NW, Ray G, et al. Bilateral osteonecrosis of the capitate: a case report. JBJS Case Connect 2021;11(4).

19. Harrington KD, Murray WR, Kountz SL, et al. Avascular necrosis of bone after renal transplantation. J Bone Joint Surg Am 1971;53(2):203–15.

20. Niesten JA, Verhaar JA. Idiopathic avascular necrosis of the capitate: a case report and a review of the literature. Hand Surg 2002;7(1):159e161.

21. De Smet L, Willemen D, Kimpe E, et al. Nontraumatic osteonecrosis of the capitate bone associated with gout. Ann Chir Main Memb Super 1993;12:210–2.

22. Newman JH, Watt I. Avascular necrosis of the capitate and dorsal dorsi-flexion instability. Hand 1980;12(2):176–8.

23. Wounlund J, Lohmann M. Aseptic necrosis of the capitate secondary to Gaucher's disease: a case report. J Hand Surg Br 1989;14:336–7.

24. Kadar A, Elhassan B, Moran SL. Manifestations of Mucolipidosis III in the hand: avascular necrosis of multiple carpal bones. J Hand Surg Eur 2017;42(6):645–6.

25. Jonsson G. Aseptic bone necrosis of the Os Capitatum (Os Magnum). Acta Radiol 1942;23(06):562–4.

26. Bolton-Maggs BG, Helal BH, Revell PA. Bilateral avascular necrosis of the capitate. A case report and a review of the literature. J Hand Surg Eur 1984;66(B4):557–9.

27. Vander Grend R, Dell PC, Glowczewskie F, et al. Intraosseous blood supply of the capitate and its correlation with aseptic necrosis. J Hand Surg Am 1984;9(5):677–83.

28. Murakami H, Nishida J, Ehara S, et al. Revascularization of avascular necrosis of the capitate bone. AJR Am J Roentgenol 2002;179(3):664–6.

29. Kadar A, Morsy M, Sur YJ, et al. The vascular anatomy of the capitate: new discoveries using microcomputed tomography imaging. J Hand Surg Am 2017;42(2):78–86.

30. Kadar A, Morsy M, Sur YJ, et al. Capitate fractures: a review of 53 patients. J Hand Surg 2016;41(10):e359ee366.

31. Ansari MT, Janardhanan R. Mid-carpal joint sparing procedure for idiopathic avascular necrosis of capitate. J Wrist Surg 2021;10(5):430–5.

32. Arcalis Arce A, Pedemonte Jansana JP, Massons Albareda JM. Idiopathic necrosis of the capitate. Acta Orthop Belg 1996;62(1):46–8.

33. Lapinsky AS, Mack GR. Avascular necrosis of the capitate: a case report. J Hand Surg Am 1992;17(6):1090–2.

34. Bekele W, Escobedo E, Allen R. Avascular necrosis of the capitate. J Radiol Case Rep 2011;5(6):31–6.

35. Shimizu T, Omokawa S, del Piñal F, et al. Arthroscopic partial capitate resection for type Ia avascular necrosis: a short-term outcome analysis. J Hand Surg Am 2015;40(12):2393–400.

36. Athlani L, Granero J, Dap F, et al. Avascular necrosis of the capitate: case series of five patients and review of literature. J Hand Surg Eur 2019;44(7):702–7.

37. Humphrey CS, Izadi KD, Esposito PW. Case reports: osteonecrosis of the capitate: a pediatric case report. Clin Orthop Relat Res 2006;447:256–9.

38. Kimmel RB, O'Brien ET. Surgical treatment of avascular necrosis of the proximal pole of the capitate—Case report. J Hand Surg Am 1982;7:284–6.

39. Jafari D, Shariatzadeh H, Nabi R. Capitate osteonecrosis: a pediatric case report. Shafa Ortho J 2017;4(2):e10100.

40. Ichchou L, Amine B, Hajjaj-Hassouni N. Idiopathic avascular necrosis of the capitate bone: a new case report. Clin Rheumatol 2008;27(Suppl 2):S47–50.

41. Imai S, Uenaka K, Matsusue Y. Idiopathic necrosis of the capitate treated by vascularized bone graft

based on the 2, 3 intercompartmental supraretinac-ular artery. J Hand Surg Eur 2014;39(3):322–3.

42. Usami S, Kawahara S, Inami K. Vascularized second metacarpal bone graft for the treatment of idiopathic osteonecrosis of the capitate. Hand (N Y). 2020; 15(1):NP22–5.

43. Burger H, Muller EJ, Kalicke T. Avascular necrosis of the capitate in athletes [in German]. Sportverletz Sportschaden 2006;20(2):91e95.

44. Kazmers NH, Rozell JC, Rumball KM, et al. Medial femoral condyle microvascular bone transfer as a treatment for capitate avascular necrosis: surgical technique and case report. J Hand Surg Am 2017; 42(10):841.e1–6.

45. Higgins JP, Bürger HK. Osteochondral flaps from the distal femur: expanding applications, harvest sites, and indications. J Reconstr Microsurg 2014; 30(7):483–90.

46. Lowry WE Jr, Cord SA. Traumatic avascular necrosis of the capitate bone-case report. J Hand Surg Am 1981;6(3):245–8.

47. Whiting J, Rotman MB. Scaphocapitolunate arthrod-esis for idiopathic avascular necrosis of the capitate: a case report. J Hand Surg Am 2002;27(4):692–6.

48. Leonard M, Mullett H. Posterior interosseous neurec-tomy for extensive idiopathic avascular necrosis of the capitate in an adolescent. J Hand Surg Eur 2012;37(6):582–3.

49. Por YC, Chew WY, Tsou IY. Avascular necrosis of the triquetrum: a case report. Hand Surg 2005;10(1): 91–4.

50. Albtoush OM, Esmadi M, Al-Omari MH. Cystic avas-cular necrosis of the triquetrum. Clin Imaging 2013; 37(2):393–7.

51. Amsallem L, Serane J, Zbili D, et al. Idiopathic bilat-eral lunate and triquetrum avascular necrosis: a case report. Hand Surg Rehabil 2016;35(5):367–70.

52. Ovadja ZN, Snel CY, Lapid O, et al. Avascular necro-sis with cystic changes in the triquetrum after trauma in combination with heavy smoking and local corti-costeroid injection. J Hand Microsurg 2020; 12(suppl S1):S58–60.

53. García-López A, Cardoso Z, Ortega L. Avascular necrosis of trapezium bone: a case report. J Hand Surg Am 2002;27(4):704e706.

54. Petsatodis E, Ditsios K, Konstantinou P, et al. A case of trapezium avascular necrosis treated conserva-tively. Case Rep Orthop 2017;2017:6936013.

55. Zafra M, Carpintero P, Cansino D. Osteonecrosis of the trapezium treated with a vascularized distal radius bone graft. J Hand Surg Am 2004;29(6): 1098e1101.

56. D'Agostino P, Townley WA, Roulot E. Bilateral avas-cular necrosis of the trapezoid. J Hand Surg Am 2011;36(10):1678e1680.

57. Sturzenegger M, Mencarelli F. Avascular necrosis of the trapezoid bone. J Hand Surg Br 1998;23(4): 550e551.

58. Hong SW, Roh YH, Gong HS, et al. Idiopathic avas-cular necrosis of trapezoid in adolescence: 3-year follow-up. J Hand Surg Am 2020;45(5):e11–6.

59. Kane P, Waryasz G, Katarincic J. Avascular necrosis of the trapezoid bone following carpometacarpal ar-throplasty. R I Med J (2013) 2014;97(3):50–2.

60. Oláh J. Bilateral aseptic necrosis of the os pisiforme. Z Orthop Ihre Grenzgeb 1968;104(4):590e591.

61. Garcia LA, Vaca JB. Avascular necrosis of the pisi-form. J Hand Surg Br 2006;31(4):453e454.

62. Match RM. Nonspecific avascular necrosis of the pisiform bone: a case report. J Hand Surg Am 1980;5(4):341e342.

63. Saffar P. Remplacement du semi-lunaire par le pisi-forme: Description d'une nouvelle technique pour le traitement de la maladie de Kienbock. Ann Chir Main 1982;1:276–9.

64. Daecke W, Lorenz S, Wieloch P, et al. Vascularized os pisiform for reinforcement of the lunate in Kien-böck's disease: an average of 12 years of follow-up study. J Hand Surg Am 2005;30(5):915–22.

65. Tan Z, Xiang Z, Huang F, et al. Long-term results of vascularized os pisiform transfer for advanced Kien-böck disease after follow-up for at least 15 years: a case series. Medicine (Baltimore) 2018;97(48): e13229.

66. Peters SJ, Verstappen C, Degreef I, et al. Avascular necrosis of the hamate: three cases and review of the literature. J Wrist Surg 2014;3(4):269–74.

67. Failla JM. Osteonecrosis associated with nonunion of the hook of the hamate. Orthopedics 1993; 16(2):217–8.

68. Mazis GA, Sakellariou VI, Kokkalis ZT. Avascular ne-crosis of the hamate treated with capitohamate and lunatohamate intercarpal fusion. Orthopedics 2012; 35(3):e444–7.

69. Juon BH, Treumann TC, von Wartburg U. Avascular necrosis of the hamate—case report [in German]. Handchir Mikrochir Plast Chir 2008;40(3):201–3.

70. Tukenmez M, Percin S, Tezeren G. Aseptic necrosis of the hamate: a case report. Hand Surg 2005;10(1): 115–8.

71. Telfer JR, Evans DM, Bingham JB. Avascular necro-sis of the hamate. J Hand Surg [Br] 1994;19(3): 389–92.

UNITED STATES POSTAL SERVICE®

Statement of Ownership, Management, and Circulation
(All Periodicals Publications Except Requester Publications)

1. Publication Title	2. Publication Number	3. Filing Date
HAND CLINICS	000 – 709	9/18/2022

4. Issue Frequency	5. Number of Issues Published Annually	6. Annual Subscription Price
FEB, MAY, AUG, NOV	4	$444.00

7. Complete Mailing Address of Known Office of Publication (Not printer) (Street, city, county, state, and ZIP+4®)

ELSEVIER INC.
230 Park Avenue, Suite 800
New York, NY 10169

Contact Person
Malathi Samayan

Telephone (Include area code)
91-44-4299-4507

8. Complete Mailing Address of Headquarters or General Business Office of Publisher (Not printer)

ELSEVIER INC.
230 Park Avenue, Suite 800
New York, NY 10169

9. Full Names and Complete Mailing Addresses of Publisher, Editor, and Managing Editor (Do not leave blank)

Publisher (Name and complete mailing address)

DOLORES MELONI, ELSEVIER INC.
1600 JOHN F KENNEDY BLVD. SUITE 1800
PHILADELPHIA, PA 19103-2899

Editor (Name and complete mailing address)

Megan Ashdown, ELSEVIER INC.
1600 JOHN F KENNEDY BLVD. SUITE 1800
PHILADELPHIA, PA 19103-2899

Managing Editor (Name and complete mailing address)

PATRICK MANLEY, ELSEVIER INC.
1600 JOHN F KENNEDY BLVD. SUITE 1800
PHILADELPHIA, PA 19103-2899

10. Owner (Do not leave blank. If the publication is owned by a corporation, give the name and address of the corporation immediately followed by the names and addresses of all stockholders owning or holding 1 percent or more of the total amount of stock. If not owned by a corporation, give the names and addresses of the individual owners. If owned by a partnership or other unincorporated firm, give its name and address as well as those of each individual owner. If the publication is published by a nonprofit organization, give its name and address.)

Full Name	Complete Mailing Address
WHOLLY OWNED SUBSIDIARY OF REED/ELSEVIER, US HOLDINGS	1600 JOHN F KENNEDY BLVD. SUITE 1800 PHILADELPHIA, PA 19103-2899

11. Known Bondholders, Mortgagees, and Other Security Holders Owning or Holding 1 Percent or More of Total Amount of Bonds, Mortgages, or Other Securities. If none, check box ▸ ☐ None

Full Name	Complete Mailing Address
N/A	

12. Tax Status (For completion by nonprofit organizations authorized to mail at nonprofit rates) (Check one)
The purpose, function, and nonprofit status of this organization and the exempt status for federal income tax purposes:
☒ Has Not Changed During Preceding 12 Months
☐ Has Changed During Preceding 12 Months (Publisher must submit explanation of change with this statement)

PS Form 3526, July 2014 (Page 1 of 4 (see instructions page 4)) PSN 7530-01-000-9931 PRIVACY NOTICE: See our privacy policy on www.usps.com.

---

13. Publication Title	14. Issue Date for Circulation Data Below
HAND CLINICS	MAY 2022

15. Extent and Nature of Circulation			Average No. Copies Each Issue During Preceding 12 Months	No. Copies of Single Issue Published Nearest to Filing Date
a. Total Number of Copies (Net press run)			304	280
b. Paid Circulation (By Mail and Outside the Mail)	(1)	Mailed Outside-County Paid Subscriptions Stated on PS Form 3541 (include paid distribution above nominal rate, advertiser's proof copies, and exchange copies)	186	169
	(2)	Mailed In-County Paid Subscriptions Stated on PS Form 3541 (include paid distribution above nominal rate, advertiser's proof copies, and exchange copies)	0	0
	(3)	Paid Distribution Outside the Mails Including Sales Through Dealers and Carriers, Street Vendors, Counter Sales, and Other Paid Distribution Outside USPS®	88	82
	(4)	Paid Distribution by Other Classes of Mail Through the USPS (e.g., First-Class Mail®)	0	0
c. Total Paid Distribution (Sum of 15b (1), (2), (3), and (4))		▸	274	251
d. Free or Nominal Rate Distribution (By Mail and Outside the Mail)	(1)	Free or Nominal Rate Outside-County Copies included on PS Form 3541	13	12
	(2)	Free or Nominal Rate In-County Copies included on PS Form 3541	0	0
	(3)	Free or Nominal Rate Copies Mailed at Other Classes Through the USPS (e.g., First-Class Mail)	0	0
	(4)	Free or Nominal Rate Distribution Outside the Mail (Carriers or other means)	0	0
e. Total Free or Nominal Rate Distribution (Sum of 15d (1), (2), (3) and (4))		▸	13	12
f. Total Distribution (Sum of 15c and 15e)		▸	287	263
g. Copies not Distributed (See Instructions to Publishers #4 (page #3))		▸	17	17
h. Total (Sum of 15f and g)		▸	304	280
i. Percent Paid (15c divided by 15f times 100)		▸	95.47%	95.43%

* If you are claiming electronic copies, go to line 16 on page 3. If you are not claiming electronic copies, skip to line 17 on page 3.

16. Electronic Copy Circulation	Average No. Copies Each Issue During Preceding 12 Months	No. Copies of Single Issue Published Nearest to Filing Date
a. Paid Electronic Copies ▸		
b. Total Paid Print Copies (Line 15c) + Paid Electronic Copies (Line 16a) ▸		
c. Total Print Distribution (Line 15f) + Paid Electronic Copies (Line 16a) ▸		
d. Percent Paid (Both Print & Electronic Copies) (16b divided by 16c × 100) ▸		

☒ I certify that 50% of all my distributed copies (electronic and print) are paid above a nominal price.

17. Publication of Statement of Ownership

☒ If the publication is a general publication, publication of this statement is required. Will be printed in the November 2022 issue of this publication. ☐ Publication not required.

18. Signature and Title of Editor, Publisher, Business Manager, or Owner		Date
Malathi Samayan	*Malathi Samayan*	9/18/2022
Malathi Samayan - Distribution Controller		

I certify that all information furnished on this form is true and complete. I understand that anyone who furnishes false or misleading information on this form or who omits material or information requested on the form may be subject to criminal sanctions (including fines and imprisonment) and/or civil sanctions (including civil penalties).

PS Form 3526, July 2014 (Page 3 of 4) PRIVACY NOTICE: See our privacy policy on www.usps.com

Moving?

Make sure your subscription moves with you!

To notify us of your new address, find your **Clinics Account Number** (located on your mailing label above your name), and contact customer service at:

Email: journalscustomerservice-usa@elsevier.com

800-654-2452 (subscribers in the U.S. & Canada)
314-447-8871 (subscribers outside of the U.S. & Canada)

Fax number: 314-447-8029

Elsevier Health Sciences Division
Subscription Customer Service
3251 Riverport Lane
Maryland Heights, MO 63043

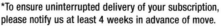
*To ensure uninterrupted delivery of your subscription, please notify us at least 4 weeks in advance of move.

ELSEVIER

Printed and bound by CPI Group (UK) Ltd, Croydon, CR0 4YY

08/05/2025

01864723-0016